ENVIRONMENT
&
HEALTH

This new series is designed to meet the growing demand for current, accessible information about the increasingly popular wellness approach to personal health. The result of a collaborative effort by a highly professional writing, editorial, and publishing team, the *Wellness* series consists of 16 volumes, each on a single topic. Each volume in this attractively produced series combines original material with carefully selected readings, relevant statistical data, and illustrations. The series objectives are to increase awareness of the value of a wellness approach to personal health and to help the reader become a more informed consumer of health-related information. Employing a critical thinking approach, each volume includes a variety of assessment tools, discusses basic concepts, suggests key questions, and provides the reader with a list of resources for further exploration.

James K. Jackson	Wellness: AIDS, STD, & Other Communicable Diseases
Richard G. Schlaadt	Wellness: Alcohol Use & Abuse
Richard G. Schlaadt	Wellness: Drugs, Society, & Behavior
Robert E. Kime	Wellness: Environment & Health
Gary Klug & Janice Lettunich	Wellness: Exercise & Physical Fitness
James D. Porterfield & Richard St. Pierre	Wellness: Healthful Aging
Robert E. Kime	Wellness: The Informed Health Consumer
Paula F. Ciesielski	Wellness: Major Chronic Diseases
Robert E. Kime	Wellness: Mental Health
Judith S. Hurley	Wellness: Nutrition & Health
Robert E. Kime	Wellness: Pregnancy, Childbirth, & Parenting
David C. Lawson	Wellness: Safety & Accident Prevention
Randall R. Cottrell	Wellness: Stress Management
Richard G. Schlaadt	Wellness: Tobacco & Health
Randall R. Cottrell	Wellness: Weight Control
Judith S. Hurley & Richard G. Schlaadt	Wellness: The Wellness Life-Style

ENVIRONMENT & HEALTH

Robert E. Kime

WELLNESS

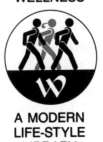

A MODERN
LIFE-STYLE
LIBRARY

The Dushkin Publishing Group, Inc./Sluice Dock, Guilford, CT 06437

AA21675

Library of Congress Catalog Card Number: 91–057936
Manufactured in the United States of America
First Edition, First Printing
ISBN: 0–87967–870–4

Library of Congress Cataloging-in-Publication Data

Kime, Robert E., Environment & Health (Wellness)
    1. Environmental health. 2. Human ecology. I. Title. II. Series.
616.98   91–057936   ISBN 0–87967–870–4

Please see page 145 for credits.

The procedures and explanations given in this publication are based on research and consultation with medical and nursing authorities. To the best of our knowledge, these procedures and explanations reflect currently accepted medical practice; nevertheless, they cannot be considered absolute and universal recommendations. For individual application, treatment suggestions must be considered in light of the individual's health, subject to a doctor's specific recommendations. The authors and the publisher disclaim responsibility for any adverse effects resulting directly or indirectly from the suggested procedures, from any undetected errors, or from the reader's misunderstanding of the text.

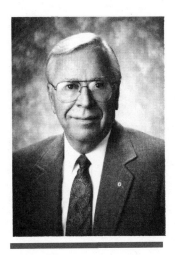

ROBERT E. KIME

Robert E. Kime, Ph.D. (The Ohio State University), is Professor Emeritus at the University of Oregon. A teacher of teachers for the past 35 years, he has specialized in the areas of consumer health, mental health, and human sexuality. His first book, *Health: A Consumer's Dilemma* (1970), was notable for being one of the first to discuss the specific health hazards posed by the questionable practices of fraudulent health providers.

WELLNESS:
A Modern Life-Style Library

General Editors
Robert E. Kime, Ph.D.
Richard G. Schlaadt, Ed.D.

Authors
Paula F. Ciesielski, M.D.
Randall R. Cottrell, Ed.D.
Judith S. Hurley, M.S., R.D.
James K. Jackson, M.D.
Robert E. Kime, Ph.D.
Gary A. Klug, Ph.D.
David C. Lawson, Ph.D.
Janice Lettunich, M.S.
James D. Porterfield
Richard St. Pierre, Ph.D.
Richard G. Schlaadt, Ed.D.

Developmental Staff
Irving Rockwood, Program Manager
Paula Edelson, Series Editor
Elsa Van Bergen, Developmental Editor
Wendy Connal, Administrative Assistant
Jason J. Marchi, Editorial Assistant

Editing Staff
John S. L. Holland, Managing Editor
Janet M. Jamilkowski, Copy Editor
Diane Barker, Editorial Assistant
Mary L. Strieff, Art Editor
Robert Reynolds, Illustrator

Production and Design Staff
Brenda S. Filley, Production Manager
Whit Vye, Cover Design and Logo
Jeremiah B. Lighter, Text Design
Libra Ann Cusack, Typesetting Supervisor
Charles Vitelli, Designer
Meredith Scheld, Graphics Assistant
Steve Shumaker, Graphics Assistant
Lara M. Johnson, Graphics Assistant
Juliana Arbo, Typesetter
Richard Tietjen, Editorial Systems Analyst

Preface

OVER TWO DECADES have passed since the first Earth Day was celebrated. Since then, much has been accomplished, but much remains to be done. And one question looms menacingly over all: Is there enough time remaining to do the job?

Daily newscasts feature a continuing barrage of information about the destruction of rain forests, farmland, wildlife, and the ozone layer. It is estimated that the world's population increases by 3 people every second, 10,800 people every hour, 250,000 every day, and 91 million people every year. Recently, the United Nations Population Fund reported that demographers have revised upward their earlier projections of world population. Instead of stabilizing at 10.2 billion people in the year 2050, as had earlier been predicted, world population is now expected to reach as high as 14 billion before population growth stops. These and a host of other developments are a cause for genuine concern.

The good news is that many people are becoming more aware of the importance of the environment and its impact on human health. As we urge our elected officials to adopt measures that encourage practical steps such as recycling, water conservation, toxic waste management, and car pooling that will help us as a society to clean up our act, we must explore ways that we as individuals can do our part.

This is not a definitive work, but rather a place to begin. The central objective of this book is not to make you into an instant expert but to help you learn to *think critically* about the information on the environment and health with which all of us are bombarded almost daily. Only then will you be able to distinguish environmental health fact from environmental health myth, and only then will you be an informed health consumer.

I wish to acknowledge all the students that I have had in classes over the years and recognize the contributions that they have made to this book and others in this series. I am especially indebted to members of The Dushkin Publishing Group: Rick Connelly, President, for his courage in undertaking a project of this magnitude; Irving Rockwood, Program Manager, Paula Edelson, Series Editor, Elsa Van Bergen, Developmental Editor, Wendy Connal, Administrative Assistant, Jason J. Marchi, Editorial Assistant, and Carolyn Dickinson for their guidance, patience and encouragement.

Robert E. Kime
Eugene, OR

Contents

Preface   vii

1
The "Fragile" Environment
Page 1

The Origins of Ecological Concern   2
Connections and Consequences
The Dynamics of the Ecosystem   6
The Tragedy of the Commons
Playing Catch-Up: Environmental Studies   12
Elder Boom Around the World • Population Growth, Economic Development, and the Environment

2
Population
Page 16

Predicting Future Populations   16
Crucial Patterns of Growth • Too Many Mouths
Consequences of Population Density   26
Less for More   27
Rural Land: Leaving It or Raping It   29
Responsibility to the Ecosystem   31
Water: Not All That Plentiful   32
Trading Trees for Carbon
Energy and People   34
Nonrenewable Energy Sources   34
Renewable Energy Sources   35
Population Growth and Health   37

3

The Tainting of Our Air
Page 38

Noise as Air Pollution

The Leading Outdoor Air Pollutants   42

Carbon Monoxide   42

Commuter Pollution: It's Worse Inside Your Car

Carbon Dioxide   44

Sulfur Dioxide and the Problem of Acid Rain   46

Particulates   48

Ozone, Photochemical Air Pollution, and Smog   49

Chlorofluorocarbons and the Ozone Layer   50

Why No One's Safe • What You Can Do to Save the Ozone Layer

Indoor Pollution   56

Leading Indoor Pollutants   57

Houses That Hurt • Home Indoor Air Quality Checklist

Consciousness, Wellness Levels, and the Raising of Them   62

4

At Risk: Good Water
Page 64

Supply and Demand   64

What Constitutes Water Pollution?   67

Recipe for Pollution Soup

Chemicals in the Water   69

Waterborne Diseases   74

Ensuring Safe Drinking Water   75

Cleansing Waters • Home Water Purifiers: How to Make a Rational Purchase • Making a Difference: What One Person Can Do

Masses of Discards   86
Solid Waste: Where Does It All Come From?   88
Where Does It Go?   90
    Truckin' Trash
    Energy From Refuse   94
    The Past Imperfect Life of Incinerators
    Recycling   98
    Selected Successful Industrial Waste Reduction
    Efforts • The Japanese Do Garbage Better, Too
Toxic Wastes   101
    The Mechanisms of Harm   102
    Love Canal: A Toxic Waste Disaster   103
    27 Ways to Beat the Garbage Crisis

5

The Waste Stream
Page 86

What We Can Do Individually   111
    Changing Attitudes   111
    Everyday Actions   115
    Chemical Hazards in the Home
The Bigger Picture and You   119
A Plan for Action   121
    Things You Can Do to Help the Environment
Glossary   125
Notes   129
Resources   135
Index   141
Credits   145

6

Taking Steps Toward a Healthier Environment
Page 108

FIGURES

Figure 1.1 A Big Blue Marble   2
Figure 1.2 Living Conditions in the Slums of London,
          c. 1850   5
Figure 1.3 An Ecosystem   7
Figure 1.4 The Hydrologic Cycle   8
Figure 1.5 The Carbon Cycle   9
Figure 1.6 The Nitrogen Cycle   10
Figure 1.7 Desertification   15
Figure 2.1 World Population Growth, 1900–2100   19
Figure 2.2 Total Fertility Rates for the United States,
          1920–1990   20
Figure 2.3 Age Structure Pyramids for Developing and
          Developed Countries   23
Figure 2.4 World Population Growth, 1 A.D. to 2100   27
Figure 2.5 Slums and Shantytowns Near Urban Centers   30
Figure 2.6 Areas of the World Threatened by
          Desertification   31
Figure 3.1 Blackened Air in Industrial England, 1866   40
Figure 3.2 The Greenhouse Effect   45
Figure 3.3 Transformations in the Air: Smog and Acid
          Rain   47
Figure 3.4 CFCs and the Ozone Layer: Measurements
          from the 1987 Antarctic Flights   52
Figure 3.5 Sources of Indoor Air Pollution   57
Figure 3.6 Where It Hurts: Health Effects of Pollution   63
Figure 4.1 Our Water Supply: Where It Comes From   65
Figure 4.2 Our Water Supply: Where It Goes   66
Figure 4.3 Sources of Water Pollution   71
Figure 4.4 Oil Spills and Wildlife   73
Figure 4.5 A Court for King Cholera   75
Figure 4.6 Sewage Treatment Plant   78
Figure 5.1 the Throwaway Society   87
Figure 5.2 What We Throw Away: A Breakdown by
          Weight   89
Figure 5.3 A Solid Waste Energy Recovery Plant   95

Figure 5.4 Recovering Solid Waste for Reuse   101
Figure 6.1 The Future of Global Oil Consumption   109
Figure 6.2 Energy Use per Capita for Selected Countries,
          1988   110
Figure 6.3 Environmentally Friendly Packaging   113
Figure 6.4 Reclaiming Aluminum Cans   114
Figure 6.5 Energy Guide for Major Appliances   120

TABLES

Table 2.1 Doubling Time of World Population   22
Table 3.1 Common Outdoor Air Pollution Problems   55
Table 4.1 Coliform Bacteria and Water Use   76

C H A P T E R

1

The "Fragile" Environment

When we try to pick out anything by itself we find it hitched to everything else in the universe.

—John Muir

FOLLOWING ANY ECOLOGICAL disturbance, the adjective "fragile" is freely used to describe the environment. However, some experts point out that nothing could be further from the truth. [1] The environment is almost indestructible, they say, having survived ice ages, bombardments of cosmic radiation, the breakup of continents, and collisions with comets and meteors. While that may be so, the evidence is growing that this planet's resilience may have its limits. As the list of threatened species expands, this fact is fast becoming our major concern: what is fragile is the set of conditions that sustains human life on Earth. The truly endangered species is *us*!

It has taken us some time to realize that this is so. For too long, environmentalists' cries of alarm seemed to have little to do with our experience. Even when we began to hear reports of forests in Europe dying from acid rain, many of us continued to believe that "it couldn't happen here." But it can, and it is, as we are even now continuing to discover. So it is that hardly a day goes by when we do not hear some new report that arouses our concern. We hear stories about declining maple sugar production in New England, about the severity of air pollution in our major cities, and about projected increases in skin cancer deaths as a

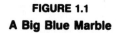

FIGURE 1.1
A Big Blue Marble

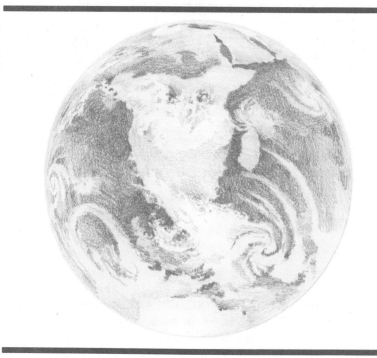

Viewing the Earth from space has dramatically changed our perception of the planet on which we live.

result of continuing damage to the ozone layer. All these hammer home the point that there *is* a relationship between the environment and our personal health and well-being. It is important to recognize that there are increasing troubles in this world we call our home. The good news is that there is also an increase in the knowledge, awareness, and desire needed to deal with the resulting challenges.

THE ORIGINS OF ECOLOGICAL CONCERN

A few years ago an informative television series for young people had as its logo a "big blue marble." It was, of course, a photo of Earth taken from space, the predominant blueness of its oceans

(continued on p. 4)

Connections and Consequences

The world's worst ecological disaster made human life possible. Two billion years ago, the tiny organisms that dominated Earth's primordial oceans dumped huge amounts of toxic waste into their environment. Eventually it killed them, along with much of the other life on the planet. That deadly substance was oxygen.

The ability of simple bacteria to remake the entire atmosphere is a striking illustration of a new view of the planet Earth that has emerged in just the last decade. Using satellites to monitor ocean currents, examining tree rings and fossilized pollen for evidence of past climates and simulating the world's future climate on computers, researchers are beginning to see Earth as a much more complex, interdependent system, in which oceans, atmosphere and life all affect one another and all help shape the face of the planet.

Among the new discoveries:

■ Plant and animal life have saved Earth from a fate similar to Venus's "runaway" greenhouse effect.

■ Ocean plankton may play a crucial role in regulating global climate.

■ Sudden shifts in currents such as the Gulf Stream can trigger mini ice ages that last for centuries.

■ Tiny fluctuations in the Earth's orbit, augmented by changes in the proportions of atmospheric gases, control the advance and retreat of glaciers. . . .

The crucial question that scientists must now answer is how the Earth's machinery will react to the monkey wrenches that humans have thrown into the works. [Humankind's] changes may be small compared with what the Earth has endured so far, but they are coming at an unprecedented pace. Power plants that instantly turn 100-million-year-old coal deposits into atmospheric gases and bulldozers that plow tropical rain forest into grazing land may not threaten the existence of the planet—but they could alter the environment for decades or centuries. Even a few degrees'

change in the average temperature of the planet could make Iowa a desert and Alberta a breadbasket, and raise sea levels enough to flood Florida and the Caribbean islands.

Although new studies reaffirm the seriousness of these threats, they offer a perspective that is seldom heard amid all the gloom-and-doom-saying of recent years. For one thing, swings in climate are natural, part of the self-correcting mechanisms that have evolved with the spread of life over the face of the planet. The machinery that interconnects life and Earth includes many gears and levers that act like a governor on an engine, stabilizing and even countering new changes over the long run. Despite bombardments from comets, fluctuations in the amount of sunlight reaching the Earth and the breakup of continents, "the Earth has protected life more than 3 billion years," says Michael McElroy, a planetary scientist at Harvard University.

Before the exact consequences of recent human activity can be predicted, however, scientists will need a precise understanding of the wheels within wheels that make the Earth run. "God has designed this system that runs perfectly," says Wallace Broecker, an oceanographer at Columbia University's Lamont-Doherty Geological Observatory. "But God didn't give us a blueprint." The degree of complexity that scientists have so far discovered dwarfs what was imagined even a decade ago. Plankton in the sea exhale chemicals that affect the formation of clouds. Ocean currents such as the Gulf Stream act as a conveyor belt, transporting heat around the world and setting climate patterns that last for centuries at a stretch. Hundreds of separate chemical reactions that take place in the high reaches of the atmosphere control the rate at which man-made chemicals known as chlorofluorocarbons (CFC's) chew apart the planet's protective ozone shield.

These connections mean that a single phenomenon such as the rapid deforestation now taking place in the tropics may in time disrupt rainfall patterns thousands of miles away. Rice paddies in Asia and cattle in South America can even add to global warming. Belching cows and bacteria that live in rice paddies produce methane gas; the gas rises high into the atmosphere, adding to the thermal blanket that traps the sun's heat in the so-called greenhouse effect.

Yet complexity is also what gives the Earth its stability. The most elaborate of Earth's stabilizing systems is the complex machinery that has evolved to handle the element carbon. Carbon is the backbone of biological chemistry, the stuff of rock and, in the form of carbon dioxide, part of the chemical blanket in the atmosphere that keeps Earth warm. The carbon atoms in your teeth may at various times in the distant past have been lodged deep within molten rocks in the Earth's interior, been floating high in the atmosphere or been part of the skeleton of an ancient species of animal. . . .

Source: William F. Allman, "Rediscovering Planet Earth," *U.S. News & World Report* (31 October 1988), pp. 56–59.

mottled with white wisps of clouds and bits of land. It is this perspective that we all need to gain—a sense of how the various components of the natural and man-made worlds *interact as a whole*. There is a certain balance, and there are connections at work on our planet.

The awareness that people should live in harmony with nature is nothing new. The ancient Greeks—especially Plato and Hippocrates—observed that disease was often associated with an imbalance between human beings and the environment. The Greeks, the Romans, and the ancient Hebrews all shared a concern for personal and public sanitation that reflected an awareness of the link between our health and the environment. Some of the great aqueducts and sewers built by the Romans are still in use today. Present-day environmental protection programs and activities are an outgrowth of the public health movement begun thousands of years ago. [2]

The Industrial Revolution of the 17th and 18th centuries resulted in a decline in public health caused by overcrowding, dislocation, and environmental abuse. These problems surfaced first in Europe and then in the United States, where the end of the Revolutionary War in 1783 ushered in an era of rapid westward migration, immigration, and overcrowding of cities, especially seaports. Inadequate sanitation facilities contributed to the spread of communicable diseases, and tuberculosis became a serious problem for the first time. Cholera invaded the continent and spread inland along trade routes and even followed the Gold Rush west to California. Four epidemics, in 1832, 1850, 1866, and 1873, left thousands dead throughout the United States.

FIGURE 1.2
Living Conditions in the Slums of London, c. 1850

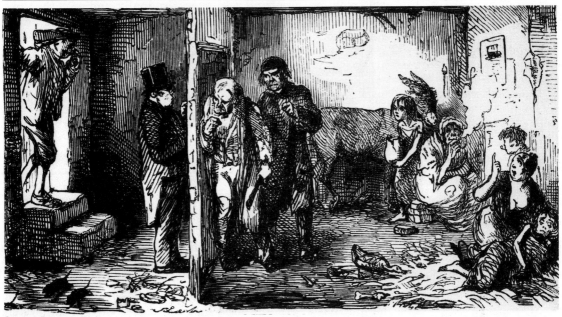

Source: Bettmann/Hulton.

During the 18th and 19th centuries, overcrowding and unsanitary conditions in urban areas contributed to the spread of communicable diseases and infant mortality.

In the midst of these terrible events, the Massachusetts legislature formed a commission in 1848 to draw up plans for a sanitary survey of the commonwealth. Issued 2 years later, the commission's report presented a plan for a health department with statewide jurisdiction. [3] This was a landmark in public health, and no less than 36 of its 50 recommendations are today accepted as standard practice. The later years of the 19th century also saw major developments in sanitary engineering and significant discoveries in the search to understand the nature and cause of disease. Louis Pasteur and Robert Koch, leading figures of this era, advanced the **germ theory of disease**, which established bacteria and other microorganisms as agents of communicable diseases. Nevertheless, raw sewage and other wastes were usually dumped into the nearest river.

Germ theory of disease: The theory that many diseases are caused by microorganisms such as bacteria, fungi, and viruses ("germs") that invade the bodies of larger organisms; this theory was proposed in the mid-19th century by the French scientist Louis Pasteur (1822–1895) and further developed by the German bacteriologist Robert Koch (1843–1910).

Exactly what was happening in that river was documented in a now-classic book, *Silent Spring,* by Rachel Carson, in 1962. [4] The years following World War II had seen further rapid population growth, economic development, and continued extensive consumption of natural resources. Gradually, and with the aid of environmental advocates such as Rachel Carson, public awareness of long-standing environmental concerns became intensified as new problems arose. People began to consider seriously predictions that human existence was threatened unless they adjusted their relationship with their environment. A new interdisciplinary science was born—**ecology,** or environmental science—to study more precisely that relationship.

THE DYNAMICS OF THE ECOSYSTEM

We share this planet with more than 2 million other species of plants and animals, most of which exist in countless **populations,** or groups of the same species occupying the same geographical area. The **ecological niche** of any given organism is a combination of the function and habitat of each of the existing species in that environment. We are all part of an **ecosystem.**

In recent years scientists have expressed concern that human activities are straining the resources of the natural system in a way that exceeds certain crucial limits called **thresholds.** When this occurs, the result is instability and, usually, environmental deterioration. Some threshold crossings are easily recognized and have foreseeable consequences. Others, though, take us completely by surprise and have uncertain long-term effects. [5]

Before we can understand the nature and effect of change on the ecosystem, we need to appreciate that living organisms exist in a state of balance with one another that is the product of a complex web of interrelationships. This balance is a delicate one; all organisms require some minimum quantity of essentials such as nutrients, light, heat, moisture, and space for survival, a requirement known as the **law of limiting factors**, and excessive change may pose a serious threat to existence. Nonetheless, change is a given in the natural world. The balance of nature is constantly being altered in response to interactions among species and environmental conditions. What is new and disturbing is an apparent increase in the rate of change that seems to outstrip the capacity of natural forces to keep pace, and is generally believed to be the result of human activities. Essential resources are renewed on our planet by a variety of cyclical mechanisms.

Ecology: The biological study of the relationship between living things and their environments; also known as environmental science.

Population(s): All the individuals from a particular species living in a given area.

Ecological niche: The functional role of a given species within an ecosystem.

Ecosystem: A dynamic community that comprises all of the living creatures and their total environment within a specified area.

Threshold(s): A point on a continuum at which additional changes in the value of one or more variables lead to rapid change in other variables.

Law of limiting factors: The biological law that the size of any population is ultimately limited by one or more environmental factors.

FIGURE 1.3
An Ecosystem

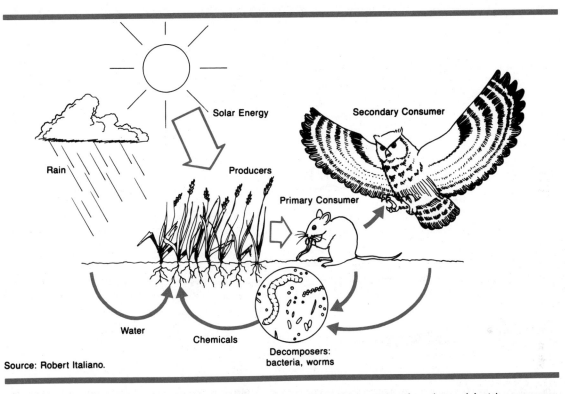

Source: Robert Italiano.

An ecosystem contains living and nonliving elements. The living elements consist of producers (plants), consumers (animals), and decomposers (bacteria, fungi, insects). The nonliving elements include an energy source (sun), chemicals (carbon, nitrogen, oxygen), and elements (wind, water).

The 3 of these most important to human wellness are the hydrologic cycle, the carbon cycle, and the nitrogen cycle.

The hydrologic cycle is the process by which water moves from the atmosphere to the earth and back into the atmosphere. **Surface water**–water found in lakes, streams, rivers, oceans, and their surrounding wetlands–is the product of a continuous process with 3 distinct stages: evaporation and transpiration, condensation and rainfall, and runoff. Each river or lake, along with the surrounding wetland area that drains into it, is part of an ecosystem called a **watershed**.

Surface water: Water found in oceans, ponds, lakes, streams, wetlands, and such, on the Earth's surface.

Watershed: The region drained by a stream, lake, or other body of water.

FIGURE 1.4
The Hydrologic Cycle

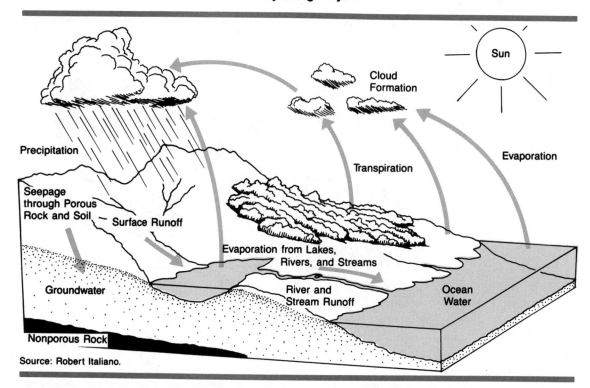

Source: Robert Italiano.

The hydrologic cycle is a natural sequence through which water circulates in the biosphere. Surface water and water from the oceans evaporate and pass into the Earth's atmosphere along with other water, used by plants, which passes into the atmosphere by transpiration. The buildup of water vapor in the atmosphere leads to cloud formation, followed by precipitation, runoff, evaporation, and transpiration in an endless cycle.

Fixation: The process by which atmospheric- or soil-based nitrogen and carbon compounds are converted into new forms usable by living organisms.

Photosynthesis: The chemical process by which green plants convert water and carbon dioxide into food using energy from sunlight.

The carbon cycle begins with the **fixation** of atmospheric carbon dioxide by means of **photosynthesis**, a process performed by plants and certain microorganisms to supply themselves with nourishment. During this process, carbon dioxide and water react to form carbohydrates, and free oxygen is simultaneously released into the atmosphere. Some of the carbohydrates are stored by the plant, and the rest are consumed as a source of energy. When the plant is consumed by an animal, some of the carbon it has fixed, or absorbed, is then used by the animal, which respires and releases carbon dioxide. The plants and animals die, they are decomposed by the action of microorganisms in the soil, and the

FIGURE 1.5
The Carbon Cycle

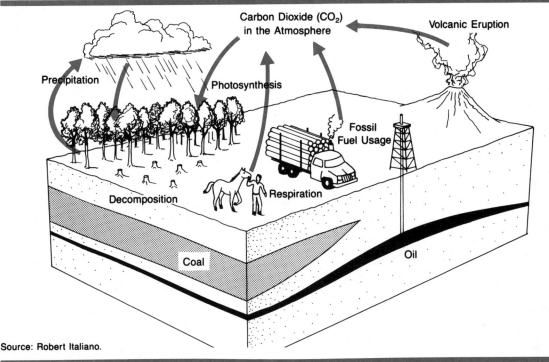

Source: Robert Italiano.

Like the hydrologic cycle, the carbon cycle is an endless sequence through which a vital element circulates in the biosphere. Atmospheric carbon returns to the earth via precipitation and by photosynthesis, the process by which plants convert water and carbon dioxide into carbon-based compounds that they use as food. Some of the carbon stored by plants is converted into coal and oil and remains in the earth for many years. Eventually, however, all carbon returns to the atmosphere via one of several routes including volcanic eruptions, respiration, the burning of fossil fuels, and the decomposition of plants, animals, and organic wastes.

carbon in their tissues is then **oxidized** and returned to the atmosphere.

The nitrogen cycle begins when atmospheric nitrogen is fixed, that is, changed into more complex nitrogen compounds by specialized organisms, such as certain bacteria and blue-green algae. Some fixation may occur as a result of lightning, sunlight, or chemical processes; however, the most efficient nitrogen fixation is carried out by biological mechanisms. Basically, the atmospheric nitrogen is changed into a **nitrate**, which is absorbed by

Oxidize(d): To combine an element or a compound with oxygen, thus converting it into an oxide.

Nitrate: The name applied to any member of two groups of compounds derived from nitric acid, known as nitric acid esters and nitric acid salts; also refers to fertilizers containing potassium nitrate or sodium nitrate.

FIGURE 1.6
The Nitrogen Cycle

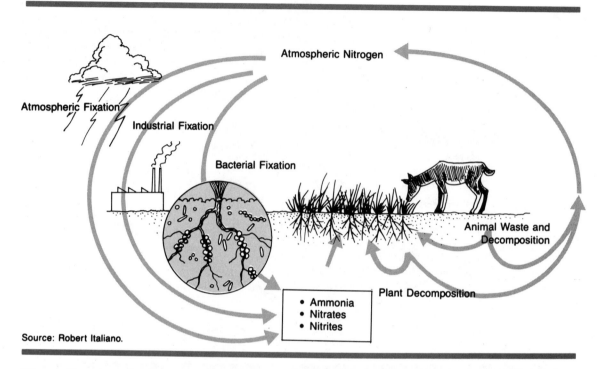

Atmospheric Nitrogen

Atmospheric Fixation

Industrial Fixation

Bacterial Fixation

Animal Waste and Decomposition

Plant Decomposition

- Ammonia
- Nitrates
- Nitrites

Source: Robert Italiano.

Nitrogen, like water and carbon, circulates in the biosphere in an endless cycle. Atmospheric nitrogen is converted into more complex nitrogen-based compounds by a process known as fixation. Fixated nitrogen in the soil (in the form of nitrates) is absorbed by plants, converted into protein, in some cases eaten by animals, then later converted into yet another class of nitrogen compounds (nitrites), and eventually released into the atmosphere as a result of bacterial action. In addition, nitrogen returns to the atmosphere as a result of the decomposition of plants, animals, and organic wastes.

Nitrite: Any of a class of compounds derived from nitrous acid; one of the most common of these is sodium nitrite, which is widely used to preserve and enhance the appearance of cured meats; various nitrites are commonly used in the manufacture of drugs, dyes, explosives, and other chemicals.

plants, eventually becoming a plant protein. The plant protein may decay when the plant dies, change to ammonia, become a **nitrite** through bacterial action, and, through further bacterial action, be released as atmospheric nitrogen. The plant protein may also be eaten by animals and become an animal protein.

Over time, the rates of transfer of energy and materials among various components of the environment have become relatively stable. But in recent years, human activity has begun to disturb these transfer rates significantly. For example, many people are aware that the consumption of huge amounts of fossil fuels by the developed nations has greatly increased during this

The Tragedy of the Commons

The tragedy of the commons develops in this way. Picture a pasture open to all. It is to be expected that each herdsman will try to keep as many cattle as possible on the commons. Such an arrangement may work reasonably satisfactorily for centuries because tribal wars, poaching, and disease keep the numbers of both man and beast well below the "carrying capacity" of the land. Finally, however, comes the day of reckoning, i.e., the day when the long-desired social stability becomes a reality. At this point, the inherent logic of the commons remorselessly generates tragedy.

As a rational being each herdsman seeks to maximize his gain. Explicitly or implicitly, more or less consciously, he asks: "What is the utility *to me* of adding one more animal to my herd?" This utility has two components:

1. A positive component, which is a function of the increment of one animal. Since the herdsman receives all the proceeds from the sale of the additional animal, the positive utility is nearly +1.

2. A negative component, which is a function of the additional overgrazing created by one more animal. But since the effects of overgrazing are shared by all the herdsmen, the negative utility for any particular decision-making herdsman is only a fraction of −1.

Adding together the component partial utilities, the rational herdsman concludes that the only sensible course for him to pursue is to add another animal to his herd. And another, and another. . . . But this is the conclusion reached by each and every rational herdsman sharing a commons. Therein is the tragedy. Each man is *locked in* to a system that compels him to increase his herd without limit—in a world that is limited. Ruin is the destination toward which all men rush, each pursuing his own best interest in a society that believes in the freedom of the commons. *Freedom in a commons brings ruin to all.*

Source: Garrett Hardin, *Science,* Vol. 162 (1968), p. 1244.

Did You Know That . . .

Chemical studies of ancient soils show that 100 million years ago, during the time of the dinosaurs, carbon dioxide levels were 4 to 10 times higher than they are today and the average temperature was 10 degrees warmer.

century. This increase, coupled with human destruction of forests and prairies, has contributed to a substantial increase in the level of carbon dioxide in the Earth's atmosphere. The quantity of the Earth's vegetation, particularly trees, is no longer sufficient to ensure that the amount of carbon dioxide consumed by photosynthesis is greater than the quantity released into the atmosphere by respiration and the burning of fossil fuels. The result is a steadily increasing level of atmospheric carbon dioxide that has potentially profound implications for our health. This is but one of many possible examples of a basic environmental rule: changes in one part of an ecosystem will cause changes in another part.

Increased awareness of the environment has in turn stimulated an awareness of how basic human social institutions and practices contribute to environmental damage. One of the best-known analyses of this linkage is Garrett Hardin's influential 1968 article, "The Tragedy of the Commons." In it, Hardin argued persuasively that there was a direct link between public ownership of property and deterioration of the environment. Property owned in common by the public, Hardin argued, is owned by no one. One result is the absence of effective limits on overuse, coupled with an incentive structure that leads inevitably to usage exceeding the property's "carrying capacity." The result is tragic, but the tragedy's origins are very much human (see "The Tragedy of the Commons" on page 11).

PLAYING CATCH-UP: ENVIRONMENTAL STUDIES

The 1980s saw an acceleration of worldwide awareness of the environment. The decade opened with publication of a 2-volume report, *The Global 2000 Report to the President of the United States: Entering the 21st Century*. This report, commissioned in 1977 by U.S. president Jimmy Carter, was the result of a joint research effort by the Department of State and the Council on Environmental Quality. The report focused on 3 major problems, which the authors identified as creating intense pressure on limited resources: population growth, the need for increased food production, and the burning of fossil fuels. [6]

As the report suggested, population growth is a critical factor in most of the political, health-related, social, and ecological crises we face today. No species can increase rampantly and uncontrollably for long without exhausting vital resources or coming up against other natural limits. Now over 5 billion, our planet's human population grows by 1 million people every 4 to 5 days, and is expected by the United Nations Population Fund to reach 6 billion by the year 2000 and to double during the next century. Ninety percent of this growth occurs in poor or newly developing countries, with the increase in the number of persons 55 and over being 3 times that of the population in general. To put it another way, not only is the Earth's human population growing rapidly, but a significant proportion of that growth (some 1.2

The world's population of persons aged 65 and older is growing much faster than the total population, reports the U.S. Bureau of the Census.

The over-65 population, currently about 290 million, is growing at 2.4% annually, compared with 1.6% for the world's total population. At its current growth rate, the world's older population could surpass 410 million by the year 2000.

Elder Boom Around the World

In many countries, even faster growth is occurring among the over-80 population. Octogenarians currently constitute 19% of the elderly population in developed countries and 11% elsewhere. By 2025, the over-80 population in some developing countries will have increased tenfold from 1975, according to the Bureau.

Already, more than half of the world's older people—54%—live in developing countries, and that proportion could reach 69% by 2025, says the Bureau. One consequence of this rapid graying of the developing world is that long-term, debilitating illness will be particularly acute in nations where preventive measures have not been taken, notes the Bureau.

In developed countries such as Sweden, West Germany, Denmark, Japan, and the United States, on the other hand, older persons may be in better general health, but their growing proportion compared with the working population could mean financial strains on social-security systems. . . .

Source: Department of Commerce, Bureau of the Census, Washington, DC 20230.

Did You Know That . . .

In 1989 12.4 percent of the U.S. population was age 65 or older.

million people a month) consists of people over the age of 55. (See "Elder Boom Around the World" above.)

One-fifth of the world's people currently do not consume enough calories to sustain them during a normal working day. Shri B. B. Vohra, an official on India's land-use board, described the situation dramatically but thoughtfully: "We may be well on the way to producing a subhuman kind of race where people do not have enough energy to deal with their problems." [7] The Washington, D.C.-based Population Crisis Committee has compiled the International Human Suffering Index, which demonstrates clear connections between high population growth and low quality of life. Population growth is a key factor in a chain, each link of which has become a focus of study, alarm, anger, and action in its own right. Depletion of resources, steadily increasing

Population Growth, Economic Development, and the Environment

The growth of human numbers and their impacts on the Earth's resources have greatly accelerated since World War II. The production of food, energy, and industrial commodities is associated with much of the deterioration of the Earth's life-support system. Between 1950 and 1986, while the world's population doubled, world grain consumption increased 2.6-fold, energy use grew 3.7-fold, economic output quadrupled, and the production of manufactured goods increased sevenfold. During the same period, U.S. production of synthetic organic chemicals, a major source of water and air pollution, increased more than ninefold. Humans now consume, directly or indirectly, about 40 percent of all the food energy potentially available on land.

Source: Global Tomorrow Coalition, *The Global Ecology Handbook: What You Can Do About the Environmental Crisis* (Boston: Beacon Press, 1990), p. 3.

quantities of solid and hazardous waste, air and water pollution—all these are inextricably connected (although we will consider each individually in the chapters ahead).

In response to growing concern about ecological problems, the United Nations established the World Commission on Environment and Development in 1983. Its 1987 report, *Our Common Future*, contained both good and bad news. On the one hand, the report noted, people are living longer, literacy is improving, and much technology is beneficial. It also identified a number of serious problems—increasing **desertification**, the role of air pollution in warming the Earth, the continuing flow of toxic substances into the water cycle and the food chain. The report concluded:

> When the century began, neither human numbers nor technology had the power radically to alter planetary systems. As the century closes, not only do vastly increased human numbers and their activities have that power, but major, unintended changes are occurring in the atmosphere, in soils, in water, among plants and animals, and in the relationships among all of these. The rate of change is outstripping the ability of scientific disciplines and our current capabilities to assess and advise. It is frustrating the attempts of political and economic institutions, which evolved in a different, more fragmented world, to adapt and cope. [8]

Desertification: The spread of desert to previously fertile areas, a process involving the rapid loss of topsoil and depletion of plant life; desertification is usually the result of the combined impact of drought and overuse and mismanagement of the land by humans.

FIGURE 1.7
Desertification

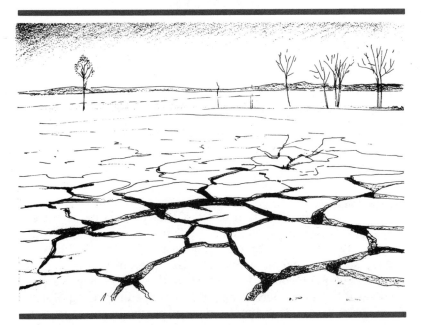

Desertification is the process whereby land that once was able to support agriculture becomes a desert as a result of poor land management or climatic change.

Perhaps so, but what this report and the work of other similar bodies have done in subsequent years is facilitate a dialogue between people and organizations. Most encouraging of all is the increase in activity at the grass-roots level. One result has been the creation of programs to tackle such problems as controlling air pollution, which contributes to respiratory disorders; reducing exposure to cancer-causing radiation; controlling industrial water pollution, which has been linked to a range of illnesses; protecting workers from chemical hazards; and preventing health problems related to noise, consumer products, and the indoor pollution of "sick buildings." In most of these efforts, as we will see, each of us can make an important difference. Human activities have the potential to tip the balance that we have been addressing. But each of us can act and live in ways that either come back to haunt us or contribute to a flourishing planet and improved personal well-being. W

Population

HUMANKIND HAS BECOME—in a blink of an eye when we contemplate 2 to 3 million years of history—the pivotal, the most significant influence in the whole ecosystem. Our present power to affect the environment comes in part from the technology we have developed but also, more simply yet perhaps more dramatically, from our numbers. It is directly due to how many of us there are, and to how we are grouped on the planet, that waters flood or waters are polluted, that the greenhouse effect builds, that rain forests disappear, or that war erupts and chemical weapons are flaunted in the quest for control over energy sources. For the first time in the 4.5-billion-year history of our planet, a single species has acquired the ability to alter radically the entire world ecosystem. Human growth, if unchecked, will outrun the possibilities of providing sufficient food and water, space, and health care, among many other things. What can we do to bring human population levels more into balance with the ecosystem?

PREDICTING FUTURE POPULATIONS

In 1929 an American named Warren Thompson made a most useful contribution to the study of populations—demographics—by pointing out that human history went through a major transition in the 16th through 18th centuries when improved sanitation and medical care made death rates decline and population growth soar. Then, about 1860, births in developed countries began to fall, largely due to industrialization's impact on life-styles. [1]

(continued on p. 18)

Environmental pressures ultimately serve to inhibit the rate of growth of every species. The sum of all of them is known as *environmental resistance.* The level of environmental resistance is not constant but changes from year to year (as climate changes, for example). It is also affected by biological factors such as plant availability and animal migration. When the potential rate of population growth is balanced by the environmental resistance, *equilibrium* is reached. In the last hundred years or so we have begun to disturb the equilibrium.

Crucial Patterns of Growth

While it was once true that the natural resources were vast, large enough to support our well-being, human influence is now disproportionate. One sign of this: underdeveloped countries have traditionally put into the atmosphere only that amount of carbon dioxide that can be absorbed by plants; industrialization has seriously altered that balance, as we saw in chapter 1.

The maximum population a specific environment can support without harmfully affecting resources is called that environment's *carrying capacity.* This capacity is not a constant factor, either; it varies from region to region. For example, a wheat field has an inherent ability to support more locusts than a short-grass prairie can. Ecosystems are stable most of the time, but it is important to remember that sometimes stability is disrupted. Erratic population blooms, sudden and unanticipated bursts of growth, may occur. Grasshopper populations, for instance, generally do not grow beyond a stable carrying capacity, but history has witnessed several periods of plagues of locusts (a type of short-horned grasshopper) which devastated crops in many regions of the world.

Populations that become too large can interfere with the well-being of other populations. An overgrowth of algae, for example, significantly reduces water quality. Large flocks of blackbirds and starlings not only endanger airplanes, but they do considerable damage to agriculture and carry a fungus that causes a disease of the human respiratory tract. A large population of rats in an urban area poses a threat since the fleas they carry bring typhus and bubonic plague, both deadly diseases.

On the other hand, scientists have become increasingly alarmed at the rate at which species are disappearing—several thousand a year, to cite one estimate—due to *our* deforestation activity and destruction of vegetation through air pollution. What's really disturbing is, we don't even know how many different species there might be: field researchers discovered 10,000 species in a single tree in Peru. We don't even know how some of these plants and animals contribute to the ecosystem. Would one of the extinct species have produced a substance that could cure a type of cancer?

Did You Know That . . .

Over 2,000 years ago, northern Africa was a fertile land that supplied the expanding Roman empire with grain. Today, this region is mostly desert, and half of its own grain supplies are imported.

That second transition has been completed in parts of Europe where both low death rates and low birth rates are now the norm.

The most obvious method for predicting population growth is to graph past population size against time and then estimate how the curve will continue into the future. The problem is more complex than that description makes it appear. Political, economic, scientific, and social changes all affect population growth. In 1900 a forecaster could not have guessed that World War I would have killed millions in Europe. In 1920 few could foresee that new drugs would drastically reduce death from infectious diseases such as pneumonia. In 1950 hardly anyone predicted that many women in most developed nations would decide to bear fewer children than their mothers did. Today the difficulties confronting forecasters include war, famine (often the result of political and economic instability), and the ever-present prospect of disease, including new ones, such as the AIDS epidemic.

The predictions we now have are frightful. The principal problem, according to demographers, is that although population growth is leveling off in developed countries, there is the potential for massive population growth in the Third World. It is estimated that the people who will alter the face of the world in the next century are being born today at a rate of 2.5 per second. If this trend continues, world population may not stabilize until it reaches a point at which we may already have overshot the carrying capacity of our planet (see Figure 2.1). [2]

A useful statistic here is the total fertility rate (TFR), the total number of children a woman in a given population can be expected to bear during the course of her life if birth rates remain constant for at least one generation. There is a clear relationship between population growth and TFR. For every given population, there is a TFR known as the **replacement rate**. This is the rate at which births will approximately equal deaths, leading to **zero population growth**. For any given population, a TFR in excess of the replacement rate will result in an increase in total population. One below this level will lead to an actual decline in population.

Replacement rates vary from country to country. In the developed countries of the world, where the resources devoted to health care and public sanitation are most abundant and child mortality rates are lowest, the replacement rate is approximately 2.1. Higher infant mortality rates in many less developed countries, however, translate into a higher replacement rate, one on the order of 2.7.

Just as replacement rates vary from country to country, so do

Replacement rate: The number of births within a given population over a given period of time (birth rate) required to offset the normal number of deaths expected to occur within that same population during that same period (mortality rate).

Zero population growth (ZPG): The maintenance of a given population at a constant level so that there is no growth in its size; ZPG advocates favor limiting births by encouraging families to have no more than some specified number of children, usually 2.

FIGURE 2.1

World Population Growth, 1900–2100

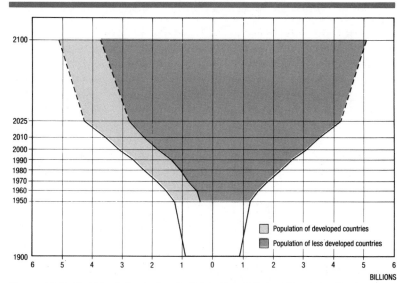

Source: N. Sadik, M.D., *Safeguarding the Future*, United Nations Population Fund.

Every year the global population grows by over 90 million. By the year 2025 another 3 billion people will have been added to the planet. Most of these people will be born in the developing world.

fertility rates. The greatest difference is that between TFRs in the developed and the less developed countries. In 1984 in the less developed countries, for example, the average TFR was 4.4, a rate at which total population will double in every generation. By contrast, the TFR in the developed nations at that time was approximately 2.0. Sub-Saharan Africa, the poorest region of the world, is experiencing population growth of 3.2 percent annually, which will bring the total population of the region to 2 billion people by 2100. [3] For a variety of cultural reasons, there is very little effective family planning in many less developed countries. In 1984 only 10 percent of the married women in Africa of reproductive age (15–49) were using contraceptives. One reason for this is the high infant mortality rate in most African countries. High infant mortality rates, coupled with the need to ensure an adequate number of children to care for them in their

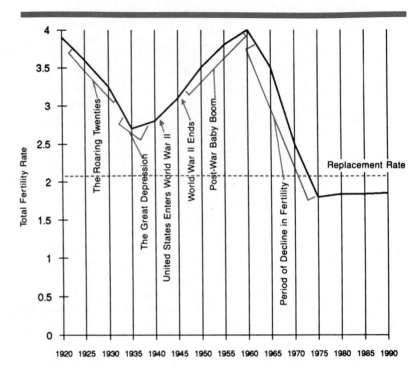

FIGURE 2.2
Total Fertility Rates for the United States, 1920–1990

Source: U.S. Department of Commerce, Bureau of the Census, 1990.

The decline in the total fertility rate for the United States may be partially explained by the development and accessibility of birth control devices and the increase in the number of women in the work force.

old age, mean that many African parents find it desirable, even necessary, to have relatively large families. Traditionally, in fact, the "desired" family size in Kenya has been an average of 7 children per family. [4]

The situation in the less developed regions of the world contrasts dramatically with that in the most developed countries, including the United States. As Figure 2.2 shows, with the sole exception of the 20-year period from 1940 to 1960 (the "baby boom" era), the total fertility rate in this country has declined steadily throughout the past 70 years. By the early 1970s, it had fallen below the replacement level, a point at which it remains today despite a recent modest upsurge in births. One consequence of this is that most current population projections for the United States forecast a decline in total population unless current trends are offset by an increase in immigration.

Another way of comparing population trends in the developed and less developed worlds is to examine the age distribution of the population in these regions, as shown in Figure 2.3. The differences in the two groups are immediately apparent. In the developed regions, where there is relatively little difference in size among the various age groups, the "population pyramid" is more like a column with a nearly equal number of people falling into each category. As a result, the number of older people in these populations nearly equals the number of younger people. The number of children may, in fact, be less than the total number of retirees, and the proportion of the population of child-bearing age is relatively small.

In contrast, the figure for the developing regions depicts a much different situation. Here the largest segment of the population falls into the younger age groups. Children far outnumber senior citizens, and people of child-bearing age constitute a large and growing proportion of the total population. In the absence of preventive measures, such populations can be expected to continue to grow at a substantial rate.

Such factors must be taken into account in any attempt to forecast world population growth. Another is the concept of **doubling time**, the interval in which a given population can be expected to double in size. As Table 2.1 shows, this interval has decreased significantly over the course of human history. During the period from 8000 B.C. to A.D. 1650, for example, the doubling time was approximately 1,500 years. In contrast, the most recent doubling, from 2 billion to 4 billion people, required only 36 years (from 1930 to 1975), and the current projected doubling time in most of the less developed regions of the world ranges from 20 to 40 years (see Figure 2.4). To put it another way, it required an interval from the beginning of human history until the mid-17th century for the world population to reach 1 billion people. Adding the second billion took another 80 years. The latest billion was added in only 13 years. [5]

What does all this mean for the future? This, of course, is a difficult question. Given the uncertainties involved, it is always easier to see where we have been than to predict where we are going. It is clear, however, that the current trends are ominous. Not only has the world population been increasing steadily but the rate of increase has increased. Given this, future increases

Doubling time: The interval required for a given population to double in size.

Table 2.1 Doubling Time of World Population

Date	Estimated Human Population	Doubling Time (in years)
8000 B.C.	5 million	1500
1650 A.D.	500 million	200
1850 A.D.	1 billion	80
1930 A.D.	2 billion	45
1975 A.D.	4 billion	36

Source: A. Nadavukaren, *Man and the Environment: A Health Perspective* 3d Edition (Prospect Heights, IL: Waveland Press, 1990), p. 47.

A population's doubling time is the time required for it to double in size. As this table shows, the doubling time of the world's human population has decreased significantly in this century.

are inevitable. The only questions are how large these will be and at what point world population will eventually stabilize. Three possible scenarios are depicted in Figure 2.5.

The key point here is that world population will eventually stabilize.

If the Earth were infinitely large, the human population might possibly continue to increase indefinitely. But our planet and its resources are finite. At some point, therefore, population growth must eventually stop. Perhaps the 2 most important questions in demography are (1) when will this occur? and (2) what will be the population at that time?

If, by some miracle, worldwide birth rates were today reduced to the replacement level, the human population would nevertheless continue to increase. Given the current number of people of child-bearing age, it is unlikely this growth would stop until world population had roughly doubled from its present level. In any event, no one expects birth rates to drop to their replacement levels overnight, especially in less developed countries where there is a disproportionately large number of women in the reproductive age group and where religion joins other cultural factors as a great obstacle to population control. In some countries—especially Mexico, Kenya, and the Philippines—religious groups have fought against any type of family-planning efforts. Others have done the same in Iran, Egypt, and Pakistan. [6] The obstacles to birth-control efforts in the Third World are

FIGURE 2.3
Age Structure Pyramids for Developing and Developed Countries

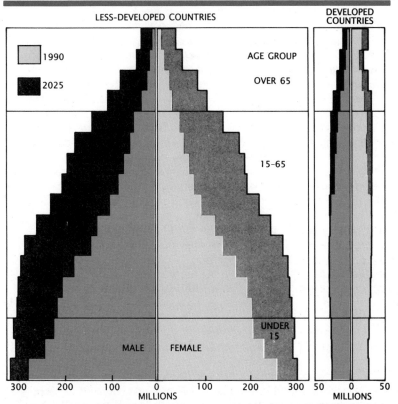

LESS-DEVELOPED COUNTRIES

DEVELOPED COUNTRIES

1990

2025

AGE GROUP

OVER 65

15-65

UNDER 15

MALE   FEMALE

300   200   100   0   100   200   300   50   0   50
MILLIONS   MILLIONS

Source: *Scientific American*, September 1989, p. 122; data from Department of Economic and Social Affairs, United Nations.

As the above graph shows, people in the younger age groups—those of child-bearing age and below—constitute a much larger proportion of the population of less developed countries (LDCs) than is true for developed nations such as the United States. Because of this, most LDCs will continue to experience rapid population growth for at least the next 2–3 decades.

Did You Know That . . .

In 1990, the median age in the United States was 32.4 years. That means that half the population was younger than this age, and half the population was older.

many. They include not only religious objections but a general unwillingness on the part of governments worldwide to allocate resources for the development of viable birth-control technology. Birth control, it seems, has a hard time competing for scarce public dollars with other more "pressing" needs such as national defense. It seems likely, therefore, that the key to defusing the

(continued on p. 26)

Too Many Mouths

Close to the Zócalo, Mexico City's great central square, lies the barrio of Morelos, a vast warren of dusty pot-holed streets and narrow entryways. The passages lead to a gloomy world. On each side of a roofless patio is a ten-room jumble. Each room holds a family; each family averages five people. The only bathrooms—two to serve 100 people—are located at the back of the patio. The odor of grease and sewage permeates the air. Flies buzz relentlessly. The people who live here are considered lucky.

In the shantytowns on Mexico City's outskirts, tens of thousands of people shelter in huts made of cardboard with aluminum roofs. There is no running water and no sanitation. The stench is overpowering: garbage and human waste heap up in piles. Rats roam freely, like stray domestic animals.

To the more privileged, those scenes look like a science-fiction vision of civilization's breakdown, perhaps after a nuclear war. In fact, Mexico City has been described as the anteroom to an ecological Hiroshima. With 20 million residents—up from 9 million only 20 years ago—the Mexican capital is considered the most populous urban center on earth. Mexico City has been struck not by military weapons but by a population bomb.

Ultimately no problem may be more threatening to the earth's environment than the proliferation of the human species. Today the planet holds more than 5 billion people. During the next century, world population will double, with 90% of that growth occurring in poorer, developing countries. African nations are expanding at the fastest rate. During the next 30 years, for example, the population of Kenya (annual growth rate: 4%) will jump from 23 million to 79 million; Nigeria's population (growth rate: 3%) will soar from 112 million to 274 million. Expansion is slower in Brazil, China, India and Indonesia, but in those countries the sheer size of existing populations translates into a huge increase in people.

In the poorest countries, growth rates are outstripping the national ability to provide the bare necessities—housing, fuel and food. Living trees are being chopped down for fuel, grasslands overgrazed by livestock, and croplands overplowed by desperate farmers. Horrifying images of starvation in northeastern Africa have captured world attention in the past decade. In India, according to government reports, 37% of the people cannot buy enough food to sustain themselves. Warned Shri B. B. Vohra, vice chairman of the Himachal Pradesh state land-use board in northern India: "We may be well on the way to producing a subhuman kind of race where people do not have enough energy to deal with their problems."

Prospects are so dire that some environmentalists urge the world to adopt the goal of cutting in half the earth's population growth rate during the next decade. "That means a call for a two-child family for the world as a whole," explained Lester Brown, president of the Worldwatch Institute. "In some countries there may be a need to set a goal of one child per family." That is a daunting challenge. During the past decade, many of the world's poor nations condemned the notion of family planning as an imperialist and racist scheme touted by the developed world. Yet today virtually all Third World countries are committed to limiting population growth.

But the effort needs to be speeded up. For starters, contraceptive information and devices should be available to every man or woman on earth who wants them. According to surveys by the United Nations and other organizations, fully half the 463 million married women in developing countries (excluding China) do not want more children. Yet many have little or no access to effective methods of birth control, such as the Pill and the intrauterine device (IUD). The World Bank estimates that making birth control readily available on a global basis would require that the $3 billion now spent annually on family-planning services be increased to $8 billion by the year 2000. The increase in funds could shave projected world population from 10 billion to 8 billion over the next 60 years. However, few modern contraceptive methods are ideally suited to the daily lives of Third World citizens. Two-thirds of the 60 million users of condoms, diaphragms and sponges live in the industrialized world. Men in developing countries frequently view condoms as a threat to their masculine image; women often find diaphragms impractical since clean water for washing the device is scarce.

The most popular form of population control in developing countries is sterilization. Some 98 million women and 35 million men around the world have resorted to that permanent solution. The other current mainstay is abortion, which the Worldwatch Institute's Brown called "a reflection of unmet family-planning needs." An estimated 28 million abortions are performed in Third World nations annually, and an additional 26 million in industrial countries. About half are illegal.

New forms of birth control are desperately needed, and a few are slowly appearing. [In 1988] a French pharmaceutical firm introduced RU 486, a drug that helps induce a relatively safe miscarriage when given to a woman in the early stages of pregnancy. Another recent arrival is Norplant, steroid-filled capsules that are embedded in a woman's arm and deliver contraceptive protection for five years. The implant is approved for use in twelve countries, including China, Thailand and Indonesia.

But progress is too slow. Additional spending on contraceptive research and development is badly needed. In 1972 global spending was estimated at $74 million annually, a paltry sum compared with many Third World military budgets. The funding in 1983 was just $57 million. One reason for the decrease was the Reagan Administration's antiabortion policy. U.S. contributions to international population-assistance programs declined 20% between 1985 and 1987, to about $230 million.

Bruce Wilcox, president of the Institute for Sustainable Development, an environmental-research organization based in Palo Alto, Calif., declared that solutions to the population challenge will demand "fundamental changes in society." Ingrained cultural attitudes that promote high birthrates will have to be challenged. Many

families in poor agrarian societies, for example, see children as a source of labor and a hedge against poverty in old age. People need to be taught that with lower infant mortality, fewer offspring can provide the same measure of security. In some societies, numerous progeny are viewed as symbols of virility. In Kenya's Nyanza province, a man named Denja boasts that he has fathered 497 children.

Of all entrenched values, religion presents perhaps the greatest obstacle to population control. Roman Catholics have fought against national family-planning efforts in Mexico, Kenya and the Philippines, while Muslim fundamentalists have done the same in Iran, Egypt and Pakistan. Still, religious objections need not entirely thwart population planning. Where such resistance is encountered, vigorous campaigns should be mounted to promote natural birth-control techniques, including the rhythm method and fertility delay through breast feeding.

If there is a single key to population control in developing countries, experts agree, it lies in improving the social status of women. Third World women often have relatively few political or legal rights, and not many receive schooling that prepares them for roles outside the home. Said Robert Berg, president of the International Development Conference: "Expanding educational and employment opportunities for women is necessary for permanently addressing the population issue."

The effect of special programs for women has been demonstrated in Bangladesh. In 1975 the government launched a project in which associations of rural village women were provided with start-up loans for launching small businesses, such as making pottery, raising poultry and running grocery stores. About 123,000 women are currently enrolled in the cooperative. At weekly meetings, health-care and contraceptive information are distributed among members. An extraordinary 75% of the co-op members of childbearing age use contraceptives, while nationwide only 35% of married women practice birth control.

Ultimately, slowing the population juggernaut will depend on the ability of family-planning experts to create well-tailored programs for different societies and even for different segments of societies. But first, governments will have to raise public awareness and rally support for population control with a cohesive message about the dangers of rampant growth. India, one of the first countries to adopt a family-planning program, some 30 years ago, failed to forge a national will for the task, and the population is now growing at 2% a year.

In contrast, China has galvanized its people behind a huge population-planning effort. Still, its program demonstrates just how difficult—and risky—social tinkering can be. The nation launched its "one-family, one-child" policy in 1979. The aim: to contain population at 1.2 billion by the year 2000. In pursuit of that goal, local authorities have offered such incentives as a monthly stipend until the sole child turns 14 and better housing. Penalties for violating the policy have included dismissal from government jobs and fines of up to a year's wages for urban workers. China's effort has had some distressing consequences. Women have been coerced into having abortions, and there have been reports of female infanticide by parents determined that their one child should be a boy. Moreover, officials have acknowledged that exceptions to the one-child rule have been frequently condoned, especially in rural areas. In fact only 19% of Chinese couples have one child. Beijing has announced that the nation will miss its target: the country's projected population in the year 2000 is 1.27 billion.

Yet for all its failings, China's effort has produced results. The population growth rate, once among the highest in the world, has been slashed in half, to 1.4%. And the Chinese are determined to reduce the rate still further. The same formidable task will face other developing countries as they confront the population bomb. But confront it they must.

What Nations Should Do

1. Make birth-control information and devices available to every man and woman.
2. Expand educational and employment opportunities for women, which will stimulate their interest in family planning.
3. Where religious preferences inhibit the use of artificial contraception, provide education in natural birth-control techniques.
4. Increase funding for research and development of new methods of birth control that are easier to use or more acceptable in some cultures than current techniques.

Source: A. Toufexis, *Time* (2 January 1989), pp. 48–50.

---

world population bomb lies in increased educational opportunities coupled with birth-control efforts, including accelerated research in birth-control technology.

CONSEQUENCES OF POPULATION DENSITY

What do all the numbers mean in terms of human values and lifestyles? What do they do to the ecosystem? What would life on our planet be like if there were 2 or even 3 times as many people in the world as there are today?

FIGURE 2.4
World Population Growth, 1 A.D. to 2100

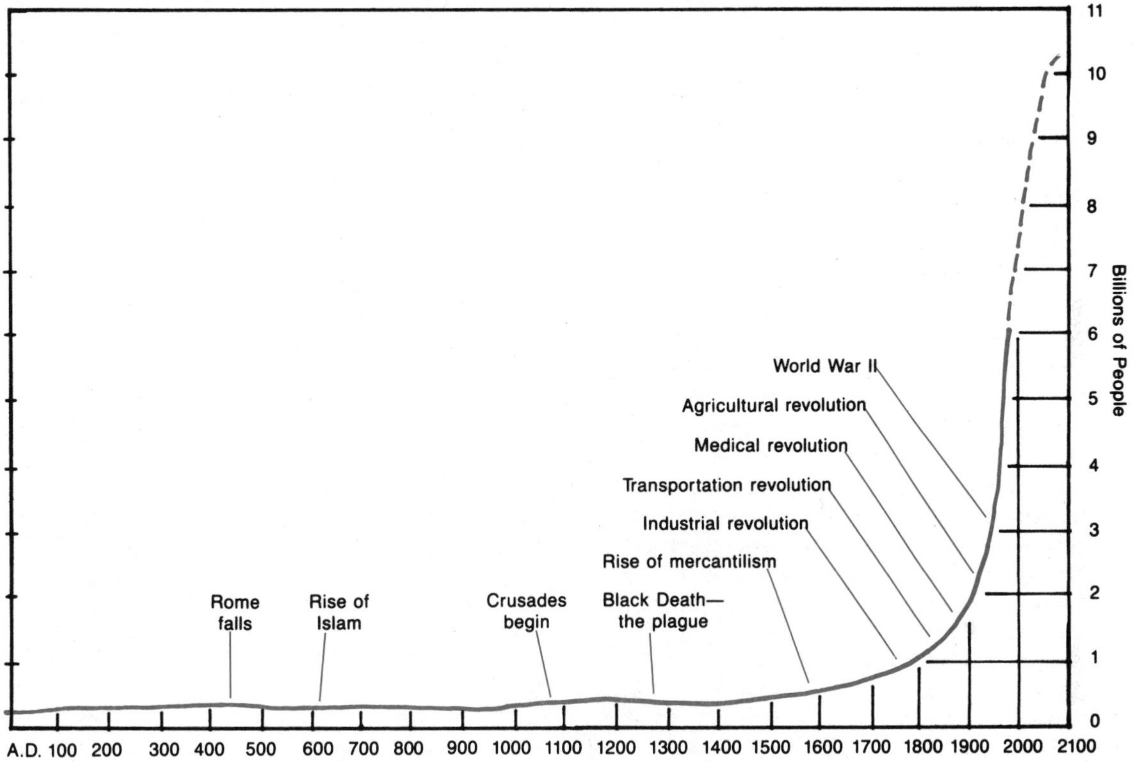

Source: Global Tomorrow Coalition, *Global Ecology Handbook* (Boston: Beacon Press, 1990), p. 25.

The world's population did not reach 1 billion people until the 19th century. In less than 250 years, the population may be 10 times that figure.

Less for More

Clearly, as the world population density increases, the prospect arises that each person's share of the available supplies of land, water, fuel, wood, metals, other resources—and especially food—will decrease. Thomas Robert Malthus, an English economist, forecast exactly such a scenario almost 200 years ago in *An Essay on the Principle of Population as It Affects the Future Improvement of Society.* [7] He believed that the world population was increasing faster than the world's supply of food and predicted a future

characterized by war, pestilence, and starvation. Always controversial, Malthus's argument has been the focus of debate since its
publication in 1798. To some he is a doomsayer, an inveterate
pessimist whose predictions have gone unfulfilled and whose
argument is based on a host of unexamined assumptions that
include a deep-seated bias against humanity. To others he is
simply a prophet who spoke before his time, a perhaps flawed but
nonetheless astute critic of the human predicament. It is a
controversy that is unlikely to go away. As Garrett Hardin once
put it, "Every year Malthus is proven wrong and is buried—only
to spring to life again before the year is out. If he is so wrong, why
can't we forget him? If he is so right, how does he happen to be so
fertile a subject for criticism?" [8]

Perhaps the simplest conclusion to be drawn from this debate
is that Malthus's underlying assumptions about the relationship
between population growth and the availability of resources
continue to concern and motivate social scientists. One recent
example of Malthus's continuing influence is a book entitled *The
Limits to Growth*. [9] Also known as the "Club of Rome Report"
(after the organization that was the primary sponsor of the
research), this 1972 work reported on the results of a Massachusetts Institute of Technology computer-based global simula-
tion. Given the credibility of the sponsoring institutions, the
report's highly pessimistic conclusions were widely publicized.
Not surprisingly, they also generated considerable controversy.
Among the critics was the at-least-equally controversial social
and political activist Lyndon LaRouche, who in 1983 published a
book-length rebuttal entitled *There Are No Limits to Growth*. [10]

But when all is said and done, it seems clear that efforts to
create computer-based models of the relationship between current population growth rates and the availability of natural
resources will continue. And such models do seem to apply to at
least some underdeveloped parts of the world. As we have seen,
most of the global population growth occurs in the world's poorest
countries. Mali, a West African country, has such inadequate
health services and nutrition that life expectancy is only 42
years, and 180 out of every 1,000 babies born there die within
their first year of life. [11] Given its current rate of population
increase, Mali would have to double its food production simply to
maintain its dismal standard of living. Yet per capita grain
production in Africa, site of catastrophic droughts, has fallen
approximately one-fifth since 1970. Similarly, declining soil and
water quality, deforestation, unsound economic practices, and
conflicts have resulted in an 8 percent drop in agricultural

productivity in Latin America. In areas like these where agriculture should provide a firm base, decreases in per capita food production always mean decreases in per capita income. [12] Some forecasters now predict that at least 65 nations will *not* be able to feed their own populations by the year 2000. [13]

Hopes for increasing food production by expanding acreage offer little promise. Most of the Earth's arable land, that which is easily cultivated, is already being farmed. Agricultural technology has a great deal to offer the world in terms of increasing production. But there are the inevitable trade-offs that will have to be made, and our willingness to make them is an issue. We will need increased energy consumption to produce fertilizers. Increased agricultural production requires the use of energy, fertilizers, pesticides, and water in ever-increasing quantities, and with these come many social and environmental costs.

Rural Land: Leaving It or Raping It
One of the results of the burgeoning population is an exodus toward urban centers. One current projection, for example, is that the population of the world's urban centers will exceed 5 billion people by 2025. [14] Billions of people will be crammed into supercities and subcities of high-rise complexes. Those will be the fortunate ones! The scenario that awaits their less fortunate neighbors is described in "Too Many Mouths" on pages 24–26. Their destiny is life in a shantytown where "garbage and human waste heap up in piles." For too many, life in such surroundings is already a sad and stressful reality. Overcrowding creates stress, which leads to both violence and illness. Researchers in the new field of psychoneuroimmunology are compiling findings that stress actually inhibits the ability of our white blood cells to fight bacteria and viruses. [15]

If present trends continue, city dwellers will increase at a rate faster than food producers. In the year 2025, 5 out of every 6 people will live in a city. [16] They will be driven there by famine and a search for a way to earn some money—only to drift into deeper poverty. Mexico City—now the most populous urban center on Earth, with 20 million persons—is expected to grow to 30 million by the year 2000. Mexico City has been described as an ecological Hiroshima—having been struck by a population bomb. But Mexico City is not alone. Of the 25 largest cities in the year 2000, only 6 are projected to be in developed countries.

The correlation between rapid population growth and poverty has been challenged as being too simplistic, yet the United Nations Food and Agricultural Organization (FAO) tells us that

Did You Know That . . .

Despite the wetlands protection provision of the 1985 Farm Act, wetlands in the United States are being destroyed at a rate of 300,000 acres per year.

FIGURE 2.5
Slums and Shantytowns Near Urban Centers

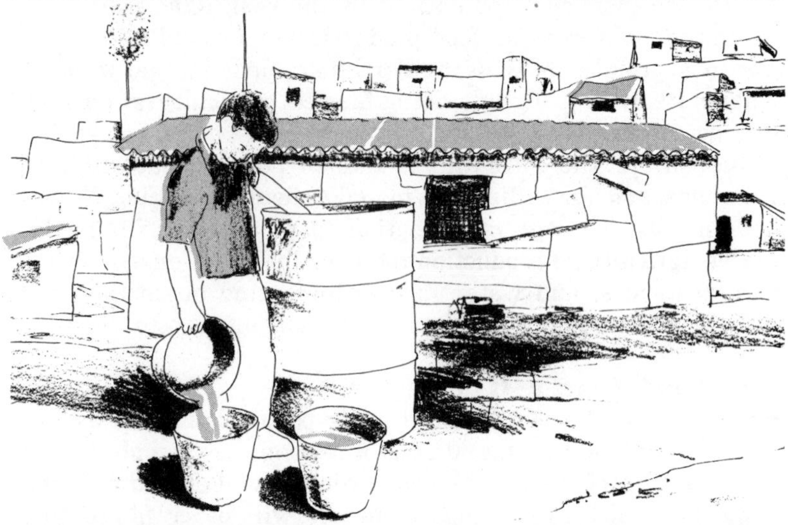

It is estimated that by the year 2000, 75 percent of Latin America's population will be urbanized. This puts a heavy demand on the supply of basic necessities such as food, energy, potable water, and shelter.

by the end of the century, more than 60 nations will be incapable of producing food sufficient to sustain their own populations; almost half the population is *already* severely malnourished. [17] The practice of slash-and-burn agriculture (felling trees and burning the land to make it arable for planting), where forests now disappear at the rate of 200 square miles a day [18] in a desperate (and we now know often futile) attempt to grow cash crops on the cleared land, has not only cost trees but pure air. (Somewhere between 23 and 43 percent of the increase in carbon dioxide comes from burning forest in developing countries.) It also results in the erosion of millions of tons of precious topsoil and a decline in water quality. As a final blow, continued over-grazing of livestock on the claimed lands encourages desertification, the process by which useful land converts to arid land or desert and is thus lost to human use. The tragic irony is not only that the conversion of forest to agricultural use often leads to economic and environmental disaster but that such attempts, even if successful, will actually result in a lower economic return

FIGURE 2.6
Areas of the World Threatened by Desertification

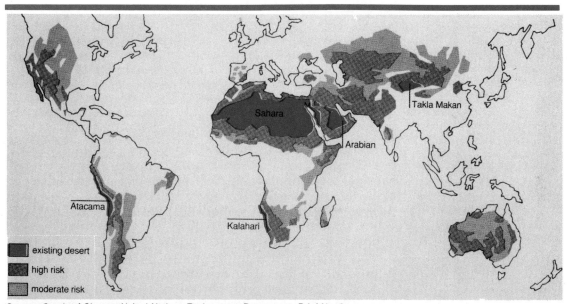

Source: *Sands of Change,* United Nations Environment Programme, Brief No. 2.

Although desertification can start almost anywhere, fertile land near the edges of existing deserts is often particularly at risk. About three-quarters of the dry lands are already desertified to some degree. The areas where the risk of desertification is highest today include parts of California, Chile, Argentina, northeast Brazil, large areas of Africa, Iraq, Pakistan, and parts of Turkey, Spain, and northwest Australia.

than if the land had been left in its original state. The authors of a major 1989 study, for example, concluded that the potential revenue from the sale of edible fruits, rubber, cocoa, and other products harvested from a 2.5-acre plot of tropical forest exceeded the value of the revenue obtained from any other agricultural use—including the sale of its timber or its value if used for grazing cattle. [19]

RESPONSIBILITY TO THE ECOSYSTEM

What is to be done? One major line of attack in the battle to preserve the delicate balance of our planet is more sensible management of the resources vital to our well-being—and to our survival. The need for such measures extends to the developed nations. For example, it was reported at the Second World Climate Conference, held in Geneva, Switzerland, in November 1990, that the United States is responsible for 24 percent of the carbon dioxide put into the Earth's atmosphere.

In response to such reports, industries and governments are beginning to act. Many industries are now taking steps to reduce their emissions of noxious substances and gases, such as chlorofluorocarbons, that contribute to the destruction of the ozone layer (see chapter 3) and pose substantial health risks for all of us. In the United States, some states now have regulations requiring reforestation following logging operations. Some local governments have begun to regulate the cutting of trees below a certain diameter, and some 30 states use tax and other financial incentives to encourage conservation or reforestation. But we have yet to grasp the total, irreversible global implications of increasing consumption of a whole range of resources—many of them in finite supply. Anne and Paul Ehrlich explain:

> While the idea that there are limits to growth seems to have been accepted with regard to population (although many still seem to think the limits are set by population density or food production at some preposterously high level), applying the concept to growth in material consumption or economic development seems to elicit consternation bordering on panic in many quarters. Part of this difficulty is that the real limits are not determined by the lack of a single, indispensable, and irreplaceable resource such as living space or fossil fuels. Rather, the limits grow out of the complex web of interactions and interdependences. . . . They are real, but they are hard to perceive and even harder to define with precision. [20]

Meanwhile, encroaching commercial development, increasing population, and individual consumption patterns are exhausting several important minerals. Zinc, copper, mercury, and lead may be depleted within 50 years at current rates of consumption. These and other similar projections suggest a need to rethink our relationship to the ecosystem.

Water: Not All That Plentiful

"You can live without oil, and you can even live without love. But you can't live without water." New York's senator Daniel Patrick Moynihan's remark points up the critical relationship of water to the human body. Quite apart from its use in industry, water is vital to human survival. Each living cell is mostly water. Blood is 90 percent water. [21] All told, the human body is approximately

. . . In the belief that the carbon dioxide emitted by U.S. power plants could be absorbed by 10 million acres of new forest, a Connecticut electric utility company decided in late 1988 to contribute $2 million towards the planting of 52 million trees over 385 square miles in Guatemala.

Trading Trees for Carbon

Concerned that its new coal-burning power plant will add significantly to global warming, Applied Energy Services Thames, a Connecticut utility company, acted on the principle that trees will absorb CO_2 from all over the world, no matter where they are planted.

According to Roger Sant, AES's chief executive, the trees planted in Guatemala will absorb at least as much CO_2 as will be emitted by the new generating plant at Uncasville, Conn. In addition to the $2 million from AES, the same amount in cash or services will be contributed by CARE, $1.2 million by the Guatemalan government, $3.6 million by the U.S. Agency for International Development, and $7.5 million by the Peace Corps. . . .

Source: J. Naar, *Design for a Livable Planet: How You Can Help Clean Up the Environment* (New York: HarperCollins, 1990), p. 127.

Did You Know That . . .

Many older houses have water pipes made of lead or of copper pipes soldered with lead. Because this lead can leach into your drinking water, the Environmental Protection Agency recommends running the water for a minute or two before drinking tap water or using it for cooking.

70 percent water. The loss of more than 15 percent of that water is usually fatal.

Because of this, it is essential that everyone have access to an adequate supply of safe drinking water. Yet this becomes increasingly difficult in the face of continued population growth. Some scientists have calculated that at present rates of use, the world supply of fresh water is adequate to support a total world population of 8 billion people—a level that current projections suggest we will reach about 2020. It is important to note that this estimate assumes that water will be available where and when it is needed. However, the world is continuously plagued by droughts and floods, and diverting water to places in need is extremely expensive and often impossible.

Current projections suggest annual per-capita water consumption in 2000 will be double the 1980 rate—more people using more water per person. In many regions, the rate of water withdrawal from rivers or underground reservoirs already exceeds the natural rate of replenishment. Water shortages are common on the mid-Atlantic seaboard, the Texas Gulf and Rio Grande regions, in lower Colorado, and in Southern California. It is estimated that worldwide about *70 percent* of the human population currently lacks a safe and dependable water supply. Overpumping of groundwater, poor land-use practices that increase runoff, and pollution of existing water supplies all reduce water availability at a time of rising need, thus posing a substantial risk to human health.

Energy and People

Population growth also contributes to potential energy shortages. The relationship between population growth and our energy supplies, however, is a complex one. On the one hand, an increase in population inevitably places further demands on available energy supplies. At the same time, the largest share of the world's energy resources is consumed by the industrialized nations rather than those with the largest populations or highest population growth rates. The United States, with less than 6 percent of the world's population and an annual population growth rate of only 0.9 percent, now consumes 25 percent of the world's energy resources. An average citizen in the United States consumes at least 12 times as much energy as one in a developing country. [22]

There are then 2 major sources of pressure on the world's energy supplies—population growth and industrialization. Both are important, and current trends in both areas suggest increasing demand for energy in the years ahead. Furthermore, the 2 factors are related; population growth creates economic needs that spur industrialization, which in turn reinforces the need for ever-greater access to energy sources. These sources are of 2 types—renewable and nonrenewable.

Nonrenewable Energy Sources

The major nonrenewable energy sources in use in the world today are coal, oil, and gas. Also known as fossil fuels, they were created by the incomplete biological decomposition of organic matter. Fossil fuels are the remnants of once living organisms that have been converted into a new form by geological processes and now contain stored solar energy. Coal, for example, originated millions of years ago in the form of plants growing in swamps. These plants died, were covered by sediment in the water, and first became peat, or partially decayed plant material, then lignite, a soft coal, and, finally, under pressure and heat, the harder bituminous and anthracite forms we know today.

Oil is the most limited of our nonrenewable energy resources; it is estimated that the world's oil wells will run dry early in the next century. Geologists believe that the last untapped U.S.

reservoir of crude oil lies beneath the Arctic National Wildlife Refuge (ANWR), an area in Alaska the size of the state of Maine and located hundreds of miles above the Arctic Circle. During the controversy over the Alaskan pipeline project in the early 1970s, when environmentalists succeeded temporarily in blocking this lucrative project, bumper stickers carrying the message "Let the Bastards Freeze in the Dark" appeared on many Alaskan vehicles. [23] People may love and value wilderness, but they also need to make a living. The proposal to tap the oil located in the ANWR has generated a similar controversy. The refuge's oil is approximately equal to a 1-year supply for the nation. If so, it is worth approximately $60 billion, including $10 billion in royalties for Alaska and the federal government. [24] Yet people all over the world, not just those in Alaska, need to understand that oil from ANWR would be a short-term solution at best, and when it's gone, it's *gone*! Natural gas supplies are similarly limited, with the result that future supplies of these 2 fuels are likely to be the product of elaborate conversion techniques. Today we are facing the fact that fossil-fuel resources took millions of years to form, yet took just a few centuries to exhaust. Developing and developed countries alike are going to have to find innovative ways to obtain energy.

Renewable Energy Sources

Obvious limits on the available supplies of fossil fuels have led to an increasing interest in renewable energy sources. Renewable energy sources are those that can be replaced or renewed rather than simply consumed. These include biomass fuel, solar energy, water power, wind power, geothermal energy and – more controversially – nuclear power (a type of energy source that escapes easy categorization).

Biomass fuel is a new name for the oldest fuel used by humans. Biomass is organic matter that can be burned directly as a fuel or converted to a more convenient form and then burned. For example, we can burn wood in a stove or first convert it to charcoal.

Firewood is the best known and most widely used biomass fuel; but in India and other places, cattle dung is burned for cooking, and peat provides heating and cooking fuel in northern countries like Scotland. Researchers on Bornholm, a Danish island, developed an energy system based on a combination of windmills and alternative fuels, pig manure and straw. Although it replaced the need for 800 tons of oil yearly, the government ultimately stopped the project as uneconomical. In a more suc-

Solar energy: Energy derived directly from the sun's rays; also refers to the direct conversion of energy from the sun to electrical energy or heat via any one of a variety of means, including liquid heat storage and photovoltaic (solar) cells.

Water power: Power derived from tapping the fall or rush of water in rivers or streams via turbines, waterwheels, or other devices; future potential sources of water power include devices to harness the power of ocean currents and waves.

Wind power: Power derived from the flow of natural air currents; the most common wind-power device is the windmill.

Geothermal energy: Energy from deep within the Earth's crust, usually in the form of heat; this energy can be tapped in a variety of ways, including wells that convert water to steam, which is then used to drive generators.

Fission: A process in which the nucleus of an atom is bombarded with neutrons so that it splits; in the cases of uranium and plutonium atoms this results in the release of enormous quantities of energy.

cessful alternative fuel experiment in Brazil, alcohol has been extracted by steadily more efficient means from sugarcane. Today 90 percent of the newer automobiles in that country run on alcohol, a cleaner burning fuel than gasoline. While satisfying the transportation needs of a growing population, this experiment has also dealt with some of the concerns over air pollution that we will examine in the next chapter.

The total amount of **solar energy** reaching the Earth's surface is tremendous. On a global scale, it is estimated that 2 weeks of solar energy is roughly equivalent to the energy stored in all known reserves of coal, oil, and natural gas. In the United States, on the average, 13 percent of the sun's original energy entering the atmosphere arrives at the ground, although the actual amount at a given site varies according to time of year and cloud cover. Physicists estimate that the average value of that 13 percent is equivalent to approximately 177 watts per square meter on a continuous basis. [25]

Another type of renewable energy source is **water power**, which involves tapping the power of rivers and streams. It has been used successfully since at least the time of the Roman Empire. Waterwheels that harness the power of falling water and convert it to mechanical energy were turning in Western Europe in the 17th century and were soon powering grain mills, sawmills, and other machinery in the United States. Today hydroelectric power plants provide about 15 percent of the total electricity produced in the United States. Although this percentage will increase somewhat in coming years, it could eventually be reduced as nuclear, solar, and geothermal sources develop.

Wind power, like solar power, has evolved over a long period—from the time of early Chinese and Persian civilizations to the present. Wind has been used to propel ships, drive mills to grind grain, pump water, and more recently to generate electricity. Winds are produced when differences in the heat of the Earth's surface create air masses with differing temperatures and densities.

Use of **geothermal energy** will become much more widespread in the western United States where natural heat flow from the Earth is relatively high. But it has an environmental price: the withdrawal of fluids and heat stored beneath the Earth's surface may undermine nearby areas, and the injection of hot wastewater may increase the potential for earthquakes.

Nuclear energy is a special case, for it has 2 basic forms, one that can be considered renewable and one that cannot. The nonrenewable form is **fission**, the form of energy associated with nuclear weapons and current nuclear reactors. Employing uranium or plutonium fuels, nuclear power plants use the heat generated by a nuclear chain reaction to produce steam, which is used to drive generators. But such power plants are controversial. They pose at least 2 major health risks. The first arises from the possibility of a nuclear accident, such as that at Chernobyl in the Soviet Union in 1986. However slight such risks given modern reactor design, and there is much controversy over this, the prospect of such incidents has made nuclear power unattractive to many people. Furthermore, the uranium "fuel" that powers fission reactors ultimately poses an extremely serious toxic-waste problem when it is spent and must be disposed of–a problem for which there is as yet no totally satisfactory solution.

The alternate form of nuclear energy is known as **fusion**. A much simpler process than fission in some respects, fusion involves a reaction in which hydrogen atoms are forced together in a way that releases enormous amounts of energy and produces no radioactive waste. Given the abundance of the basic fuel, hydrogen, fusion could be a renewable energy source. However, we have yet to devise a way in which to produce a self-sustaining and controlled fusion reaction.

POPULATION GROWTH AND HEALTH

We can see, then, that population growth is linked to a variety of problems, all of which have potential implications for our health. The increasing demand for land, food, water, and energy that accompanies population growth, coupled with the ever-present risk that the demand for these vital resources will outstrip the available supply, poses major dangers to our environment. And with these dangers come serious health risks. Poor land-use patterns caused by overpopulation increase the probability of hunger and famine. Excessive demands on water supplies threaten the health of people in many countries, while the quest for ever-increasing amounts of energy leads in turn to the increased risk of air and water pollution and other serious consequences.

We must recognize that while technology can provide us with alternatives to our present types of resources, too many of our essential resources are limited and endangered. Bringing our numbers and our resources into balance is our best hope. To do this, we must work to contain population growth and to modify our own consumption patterns. 〔W〕

Fusion: The process in which light atomic nuclei combine (fuse) to form a heavier material, as when deuterium (a hydrogen isotope) nuclei are fused to form helium; the fusion process releases enormous amounts of energy and is the means by which the energy produced in the interior of stars is generated; to date, fusion has occurred on Earth only in hydrogen-bomb explosions.

3

The Tainting of Our Air

It begins with heat: jets of coal dust and air bursting into flame at 3,500° F in the fire chambers of electric power plants; molten sulphide ores bubbling and blistering in smelter furnaces; gasoline exploding at 4,500° F under the steel cylinder heads of trucks, buses and automobiles; diesel oil, Exxon regular, bituminous coal, anthracite, lignite, the ores of nickel and copper, pyrrhotite, pentlandite, niccolite, chrysolite, burning until the heat cracks their internal electron bonds and breaks each compound into its constituents, to rise, as gases, vapor or microscopic particles, into the air.

"Precursors," chemists call them, harbingers of things to come.

Because of them, and their end products, 50,000 to 200,000 people with asthma or other lung disorders will die prematurely this year. [1]

Air pollution: The contamination of the atmosphere by substances other than water.

Toxic substances: Substances that are known to produce harmful or poisonous effects upon exposure, usually through interference with one or more of the chemical reactions that take place in living tissues.

THERE IS, it would seem, something wrong with our air. That something is **air pollution**, the contamination of the Earth's atmosphere by solid, liquid, or gaseous substances other than water. Only some of the pollutants in our air are the result of human activity. Dust and ashes from volcanoes, pollen from plants, and salt crystals from the ocean are all present in our air as a result of natural processes. There is no such thing as "pure" air.

There is, however, such a thing as "clean" air. Clean air is air that is fit for human consumption, that can be safely breathed without endangering human health. It is air that does not contain a harmful level of **toxic substances**, substances that when ingested have the potential to cause illness, physical distress, or even death.

The key words here are "harmful level." The problem is not so much that human activity has introduced new and more toxic pollutants into our atmosphere as it is the quantity of those pollutants. Carbon monoxide, hydrocarbons, nitrogen and sulfur oxides, and fine smoke and dust particles, all are being added to the Earth's atmosphere at an alarming rate as a result of human activity. So, too, are a variety of pollutants such as chlorofluorocarbons, whose most harmful effects, of which we have only recently become aware, are indirect rather than immediate.

While very few of these substances are good for us, just how much of a threat any given substance poses in any given case depends on a variety of key factors. One is quantity of the substance that is made available, also known as **dosage**. Another is the substance's level of **toxicity**. A third is the extent of exposure. There are 2 basic operating principles here that together determine the extent of the danger involved.

The first of these principles says that the amount of harm that may result from exposure to a particular substance is a function of the amount of the substance that is consumed, absorbed, or inhaled. The larger the quantity, the greater the risk of harm. Virtually all substances are potentially harmful if present in sufficiently large quantities. Taking 2 aspirin can help cure a headache; taking an entire bottle is a very bad idea. Similarly, there is for all substances a level below which any health risks involved are minimal or nonexistent. Inhaled in quantity, methane is a highly poisonous gas. At the level at which it is normally present in the Earth's atmosphere, however, it poses no health risks whatsoever. The point is that it is not sufficient to know that a given substance is present. We must also know how much.

The second basic principle says that the level of risk in any given case is a product of both the substance's potential to cause harm (its toxicity) and the level of exposure. Some substances are clearly more harmful than others. The puffer fish (or *fugu* as it is known to the Japanese, who prize its raw flesh as a delicacy) contains a poison that is 275 times deadlier than cyanide. There is no known antidote, and exposure to an extremely small dose is fatal within a period ranging from a few minutes to a few hours. The toxicity of the puffer fish poison is extremely high. For this reason, those Japanese restaurant owners who offer puffer fish to their clients take great pains to ensure that the portions of the fish that contain the toxin are removed. Despite its toxicity, the puffer fish poses a risk only to those unlucky individuals—approximately 20 a year, virtually all Japanese—whose misfortune it is to consume an improperly prepared dish of *fugu*. For the

The sources of atmospheric methane include wetlands, domestic animals, biomass burning, and the decay of landfill waste. The average methane molecule remains in the atmosphere for 12.5 years.

Dosage: The quantity of a given substance associated with a given measurable or observable effect.

Toxicity: The relative strength of a toxic substance; substances whose toxicity is high require only a small dosage to produce harmful effects.

FIGURE 3.1
Blackened Air in Industrial England, 1866

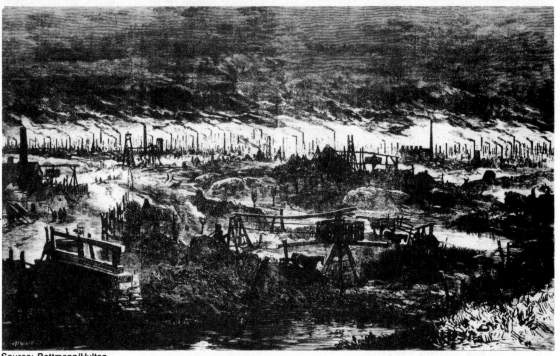

Source: Bettmann/Hulton.

Air pollution first became a serious problem during the Industrial Revolution of the 18th and 19th centuries.

rest of us, the toxin of the puffer fish poses no health risks, for our exposure is zero, and zero times any level of toxicity is zero.

In short, in order to assess the potential health effects of any substance, we must know not only its level of toxicity but the quantity in which it is present and the extent of our exposure. Only then can we accurately assess the level of risk. So it is with all potential toxins, including the harmful substances that are increasingly found in our air. Among these are gases such as carbon monoxide, complex chemical compounds, and a host of extremely small particles of solid matter.

The presence of harmful substances in our air is not a completely new phenomenon. As early as 1306, a proclamation by

(continued on p. 42)

The bulk of this chapter focuses on the substances we put into the air that have the potential to harm us. It is worthwhile to note, however, that there are other types of air pollution. One of these is noise.

Sound is simply a wave motion in air: it strikes the eardrum and vibrations are converted to messages sent to the brain. Sound does not accumulate in the environment. Ring a bell or whisper a few words to

Noise as Air Pollution

your friend, and in about a thousandth of a second the sound is gone. But sounds, especially loud ones, do affect humans, and these effects do not disappear so easily. The human ear is sensitive to a wide range of sound intensities. The softest sound that we can hear is measured as 0 dB (decibel). The highest ranges of noise, such as a rocket taking off or the noise of battle, are billions of times more powerful than the patter of raindrops on soft earth.

Noise can be defined simply as unwanted sound. Noise can interfere with our communication, diminish our hearing, and affect our health and our behavior. Current estimates are that 8 million production workers are exposed to volumes over the danger level of 80–85 dB, and over 1.5 million of them have detectable hearing loss as a result. The general level of city noise is high enough to deafen any of us, gradually, as we grow older. In the absence of such noise, hearing need not deteriorate with advancing age: inhabitants of quiet societies generally hear as well in their 70s as New Yorkers do in their 20s.

There has been recent concern that rock-and-roll music is hazardously loud—levels of 125 dB have been recorded as amplification systems are increasing in power. Such noise is at the edge of pain and is unquestionably deafening. Noise levels as high as 135 dB should *never* be experienced, even for a brief period, because the effects can be instantaneously damaging. If the noise level exceeds about 150 or 160 dB, the eardrum might be ruptured beyond repair.

Many investigators believe that loss of hearing is not the most serious consequence of excess noise. The first effects are anxiety and stress or, in extreme cases, fright. These reactions produce body changes such as increased rate of heartbeat, constriction of blood vessels, digestive spasms, and dilation of the pupils of the eyes. The long-term effects of such overstimulation are difficult to assess, but it is known that in animals it damages the heart, brain, and liver and produces emotional disturbances. The emotional effects on people are difficult to measure, but psychologists have learned that work efficiency goes down as the noise level goes up.

Did You Know That . . .

Hearing loss is usually caused by continual exposure to sounds at volumes of 80–85 decibels and above. Current estimates are that 8 million production workers in the United States are exposed to noise at this level, and that 1.5 million of them have detectable hearing loss as a result.

Edward I of England banned the burning of "sea-coales" by London craftsmen. [2] In general, however, the air was relatively pure until the Industrial Revolution of the 18th and 19th centuries, when coal burned in industrial and household furnaces and railroad locomotives blackened the air of many cities and portions of the countryside in Europe and the United States. Throughout the first half of this century, increasingly lethal winter smogs were a significant cause of death in London. It was not until 1952, when smog cost the lives of over 4,000 Londoners, that stringent and ultimately successful antipollution measures were adopted.

Then and now, the major cause of air pollution is the large-scale burning of fossil fuels. As we shall see, there are other sources of air pollution as well, and not all of these confine their effects to the air "outside." Increasingly, we must be concerned about the substances that pollute the air in our homes and offices. Experts agree: whether outdoors or in, about 60 percent of us are now breathing air that is unhealthy at least some of the time.

THE LEADING OUTDOOR AIR POLLUTANTS

Outdoor air pollution is caused by a variety of substances, some gaseous and some solid. Here we will focus on the following leading causes of outdoor air pollution: carbon monoxide, carbon dioxide, sulfur oxide, particulates, photochemical reactions, and chlorofluorocarbons (CFCs).

Carbon Monoxide

The greatest contributor to air pollution for the city dweller is **carbon monoxide (CO)**, a colorless, odorless, and tasteless gas that results when carbon is not oxidized or burned up completely. In most cities, over 90 percent of the carbon monoxide in the air comes from the incomplete combustion of carbon in motor fuels—automobile exhaust. Tobacco smoke is the second most common source of carbon monoxide. A smoker will absorb 2 times more carbon monoxide daily than a nonsmoker, and a smoker driving in busy traffic may be exposed to much more carbon monoxide than would be considered toxic. In some parts of the country, wood stoves are also an important source of carbon monoxide.

Carbon monoxide interferes with the blood's ability to carry oxygen to the brain, heart, and other vital organs. It does this because it readily combines with hemoglobin, forming carboxyhemoglobin, a relatively stable compound that, once formed,

Carbon monoxide (CO): A colorless, odorless gas formed as a by-product during the incomplete combustion of fossil fuels; it is also found in coal gas and in the exhaust of internal-combustion engines.

El Monte, Calif.—Here's yet another reason to curse traffic jams. When you're stuck in one, you breathe up to four times the air pollution you'd inhale if you were, say, sitting under a tree in your backyard.

Researchers at California's South Coast Air Quality Management District discovered this unhappy fact by installing monitors in the cars of 140 Los Angeles commuters.

Commuter Pollution: It's Worse Inside Your Car

Most air pollution studies have focused on outdoor measurements, but people usually spend only two to five hours of each day outdoors. In Los Angeles, many people spend at least that much time in their cars, leading researchers to wonder just how much pollution they breathe in there.

Of the 16 pollutants measured, seven of the most dangerous were two to four times higher in cars than at outdoor monitoring stations. For most, average concentrations fell below levels generally considered harmful. But in a few cars, chemicals such as carbon monoxide and benzene were well above acceptable levels.

Carbon monoxide exceeded state limits in 3 percent of the cars sampled. In one car, the concentration was more than twice the limit. Prolonged exposure to such amounts can cause headaches and worsen heart disease.

Based on measurements of the total benzene in the air, researchers have estimated that Los Angeles residents run a one in 10,000 risk of getting cancer from the chemical. This study shows that exposure while commuting accounts for 15 percent of that risk. Ditas Shikiya, an air quality specialist who led the study, says the benzene problem may be even worse in other urban areas, because gasoline pumps in California are equipped with nozzles that limit the chemical's release.

As far as the researchers can tell, there doesn't seem to be much you can do to clean up the air in your car. Neither rolling up the windows nor closing vents helped much, although cars less than six years old and those traveling more than 30 MPH took in slightly fewer toxins.

Source: *Hippocrates*, September/October 1989, p. 10.

Did You Know That . . .

In 1988 there were approximately 188.9 million registered motor vehicles in the United States. These traveled an estimated 2 trillion miles and consumed almost 130 billion gallons of fuel.

prevents the hemoglobin from combining with and distributing oxygen. The result is asphyxiation. Laboratory tests have shown that levels of carbon monoxide such as those presently found in some major cities can produce impairment of vision and decreased ability to perceive and respond to one's environment. Investigators have found higher than normal carboxyhemoglobin levels in individuals who have had automobile accidents. However, even though heavy freeway traffic can raise carbon monoxide levels to 60 milligrams or more per cubic meter of air—the level at which skills are impaired—we still do not have enough evidence to confirm carbon monoxide as a cause of traffic accidents. [3]

Carbon Dioxide

Like carbon monoxide, carbon dioxide (CO_2) is an odorless, colorless gas that is a by-product of combustion (or burning) involving a carbon-based fuel such as coal, wood, or oil. However, whereas incomplete combustion (oxidation) leads to the creation of carbon monoxide, carbon dioxide is formed when the oxidation process is carried to completion. Carbon dioxide is also a normal by-product of the respiratory process and photosynthesis, exists naturally in the Earth's atmosphere, and has a variety of practical uses. In its solid form, known as "dry ice," it is used to preserve foods. As a gas, it is used to carbonate beverages. It is approximately 1.5 times heavier than air and neither burns nor supports combustion.

Unlike carbon monoxide and many other pollutants, carbon dioxide is not toxic. Furthermore, it constitutes a relatively small proportion of the Earth's atmosphere, roughly 0.3 percent. The level of carbon dioxide in our atmosphere has nonetheless become a major concern to many scientists because of its critical contribution to the **greenhouse effect**. The greenhouse effect is so named because the carbon dioxide in the atmosphere acts like the glass in a greenhouse. The panes of glass let sunlight into the greenhouse, which is then warmed by the solar radiation. At night, the resulting heat radiates away from the building, but its progress is slowed by the glass. Because the glass reduces the rate of heat loss, the interior of the greenhouse stays relatively warm.

Like the panes of glass in a greenhouse, carbon dioxide and other gases in the Earth's atmosphere (nitrous oxide, methane, and CFCs) allow solar energy in the form of sunlight to reach and warm the Earth but slow the radiation of heat away from its surface. The greenhouse effect is a natural mechanism whose existence is essential to our survival. It has been estimated that if there were no gases in the atmosphere capable of slowing the radiation of heat away from the Earth, the temperature of its surface would drop precipitously, the oceans would freeze over, and life as we know it would be impossible. [4]

Current concerns about the greenhouse effect arise from its apparent connection to global warming. Although the evidence is

Greenhouse effect: The heating effect on the Earth caused when long-wave (infrared) radiation emitted from the Earth's surface is absorbed by trace gases (notably carbon dioxide and methane) in the atmosphere and partially radiated back to the Earth's surface.

FIGURE 3.2
The Greenhouse Effect

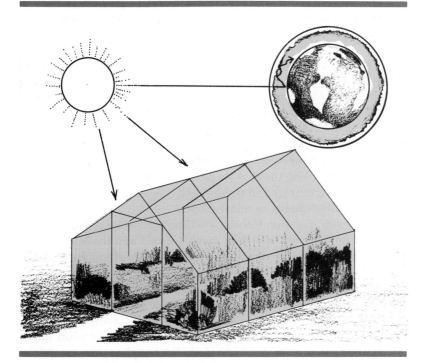

Carbon dioxide and other gases in the Earth's atmosphere act like the glass in a greenhouse, trapping much of the heat that is radiated from the Earth's surface.

not yet definitive, many scientists are convinced that the Earth is warming. For example, Philip Jones and Tom Wigley, climatologists at the University of East Anglia in Norwich, England, recently reported on the results of a 10-year analysis of global temperature trends. They concluded that "our work shows conclusively that the world's climate, although highly variable over periods of decades or less, has become generally warmer during the past century." [5] Other scientists have reported similar results, and these reports have fueled numerous alarming predictions. Writing in the April 1989 issue of *Scientific American*, Richard Houghton and George Woodwell of the Woods Hole Research Center warned emphatically,

The world is warming. Climatic zones are shifting. Glaciers are melting. Sea level is rising.... The warming, rapid now, may become even more rapid as a result of the warming itself, and it will continue into the indefinite future.... A rapid and continuous warming will not only be destructive to agriculture but also lead to the widespread death of forest trees, uncertainty in water supplies and the flooding of coastal areas. [6]

This is a grim prospect indeed, and one that, if real, is thought by many to be directly related to the buildup of carbon dioxide in our atmosphere. There is little controversy over the fact that carbon dioxide levels are increasing. [7] Researchers agree that over the past century, the amount of carbon dioxide has increased by about 25 percent, from just under 290 parts per million to just under 350 parts per million. [8] Predictions about the future vary, but there is no particular reason to believe this buildup will stop until and unless its major cause, the large-scale burning of fossil fuels, is eliminated.

The major question here is whether the 2 trends—the clearly documented increase in carbon dioxide levels and the less certain global warming trend—are in fact related. Scientists disagree on this critical point, but the evidence is strong enough to justify concern. Has the greenhouse effect begun to alter our weather? If so, how much will temperatures rise once carbon dioxide levels reach twice their current value (which some scientists predict may occur as soon as 2030)? These are among the crucial questions that remain to be answered. Although some computer models say that warming is under way, not everyone agrees. And that leaves society with a painfully familiar choice—how to act in the face of uncertainty. [9]

Sulfur Dioxide and the Problem of Acid Rain

Another modern-day environmental problem arising from air pollution is **acid rain**. Acid rain is a phenomenon that results from the workings of the atmosphere's own self-cleaning mechanism. The primary cause is an increased level of **sulfur dioxide (SO_2)** in the atmosphere generated as a by-product of the burning of fossil fuels, particularly coal. In addition, some industrial processes such as smelting contribute to the problem. As with carbon dioxide levels, the increase in SO_2 levels results almost entirely from human activity.

Like carbon dioxide, sulfur dioxide is a trace element in the Earth's atmosphere. It is estimated that the average concentration of SO_2 in the atmosphere a century ago was less than 1 part per billion. Even today in the most heavily industrialized na-

Acid rain: Rain that contains relatively high concentrations of acid-forming air pollutants, such as sulfur and nitrogen oxides; acid rain may have a pH level as low as 2.8 (on a scale that ranges from 1 to 14) as compared to normal rain's pH of 6.

Sulfur dioxide (SO_2): A colorless gas with a choking odor that is a by-product of the combustion of substances such as fossil fuels that contain sulfur; it is chiefly used in the manufacture of chemicals such as sulfuric acid.

FIGURE 3.3
Transformations in the Air: Smog and Acid Rain

Smog. Nitrogen oxides (NOx, produced by combustion processes) combine with volatile organic chemicals (VOCs, which include gasoline vapor, paint thinners, dry-cleaning fluid and many other industrial chemicals) in the presence of sunlight to form ozone, an irritating chemical that is the chief component of smog. Carbon monoxide (CO) from combustion adds to the toxic brew.

Acid rain. NOx and sulfur oxides (SOx), most of it produced by power plants burning sulfur-containing coal, react with water vapor and other naturally occurring chemicals higher in the atmosphere to form acids that fall to earth as acid rain.

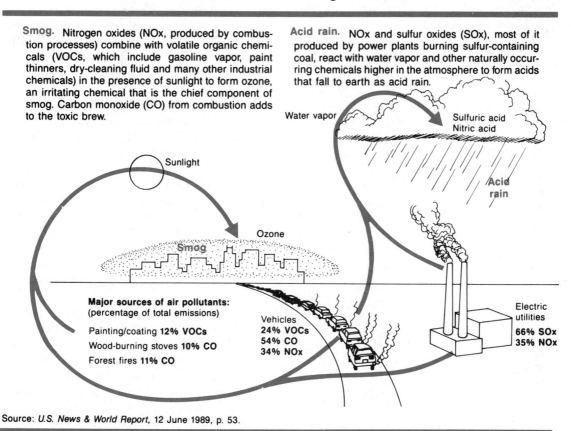

Major sources of air pollutants:
(percentage of total emissions)

Painting/coating **12% VOCs**
Wood-burning stoves **10% CO**
Forest fires **11% CO**

Vehicles
24% VOCs
54% CO
34% NOx

Electric utilities
66% SOx
35% NOx

Source: *U.S. News & World Report*, 12 June 1989, p. 53.

Although smog and acid rain have similar sources, the mechanisms which produce them are different.

tions, where the concentrations are highest, it rarely constitutes as much as 50 parts per billion. [10] Nonetheless, the increased levels of SO_2 have important environmental and health effects.

When coal is burned, most of the sulfur it contains—approximately 97 percent—is converted to SO_2 via oxidation. High concentrations of SO_2 are themselves harmful to health. They contribute to a variety of respiratory problems, including asthma, bronchitis, and emphysema. When present in sufficient quantities, SO_2 can produce a particularly harmful form of **smog**, a term coined early in this century to describe a form of combined smoke and fog. The smog that killed 4,000 Londoners in 1952 was

Smog: A dense mixture of smoke and fumes combined with fog that is formed when air pollutants (particularly exhaust from automobiles) are trapped at ground level by a temperature inversion; smog is most common in heavily urbanized or industrial areas.

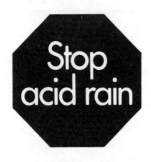

International Symbol of the Stop Acid Rain Movement

The international symbol of the Stop Acid Rain movement shown here has appeared all over the world, in many languages.

actually an SO_2 smog. Such smogs pose a special health threat because they inhibit the sweeping action of the cilia, small hairs that line our respiratory passages. The result is that the cilia are unable to remove the smog particles. Their presence irritates sensitive tissues and is particularly harmful to old people, small children, and those with chronic respiratory diseases or certain heart conditions. These and other health problems are the most immediate side effect of the burning of coal, especially coal with a high sulfuric content.

Sulfur dioxide's contribution to acid rain occurs over a longer interval. Here the primary culprit is another type of sulfur oxide, sulfur trioxide (SO_3). Sulfur trioxide is formed in 2 ways. When coal is burned, a small proportion, roughly 3 percent, of the sulfur is directly converted to SO_3. A more important source, however, is the gradual oxidation of the SO_2 that is the primary sulfur by-product of burning coal. As this occurs, the SO_2 is slowly converted to SO_3. The SO_3 in turn reacts fairly rapidly with the water vapor in the air to produce sulfuric acid (H_2SO_4). Through a similar process, nitric acid (N_2SO_3) is also formed. Highly soluble in water, the molecules of H_2SO_4 and N_2SO_3 remain suspended in the atmosphere in droplets of water until washed out of the sky in the form of rain or snow.

Only 20 years ago, acid rain was not an issue; very few people knew how much damage it could do. It affects food chains and drinking water; it can dissolve toxic elements in the soil, thus contaminating water supplies; it damages forests; it can kill off fish with amazing speed. The cause and cure of acid rain are well known. Antiquated coal-fired power plants are the primary source of sulfur dioxide. Just 50 generating stations, most located in the Midwest, account for half of the U.S. sulfur pollution. These contribute mightily to the acid rain that falls on Canada and in turn to Canadian irritation with the U.S. government for its reluctance to promulgate strong regulations. [11]

Particulates

Particulate matter: Solid or liquid particles that are suspended in the Earth's atmosphere, especially pollutants.

Particulate matter is a general term for countless particles of solids and liquids that are dispersed in our air. Many of these are generated by the burning of coal, which produces enormous quantities of soot and sulfur particles. Surface mining, refining of ores, the manufacture of metals, the grinding and spraying that accompanies construction, and automobile exhaust also release particles—perhaps in an even greater quantity than coal combustion. [12] Large particles are relatively harmless to humans, who trap them in the cilia and mucus of nasal passages. Smaller particles—up to 5 micrometers—escape these filters, as do pollutants breathed in through the mouth (by joggers, for example, or children playing).

Two types of particulates that are especially harmful are lead and asbestos. Lead is a cumulative poison, a serious health risk to children and the unborn. It can damage the blood system, kidneys, and the nervous and reproductive systems. Some 90 percent of airborne lead comes from automobiles that burn leaded gasoline. Thanks to federal regulations requiring unleaded gasoline in newer automobiles, the levels of airborne lead in most major U.S. cities are today lower than they were 10 or 15 years ago. Airborne lead remains a potentially major problem, however, because of its toxicity. From 30 to 50 percent of all inhaled lead particles reach the bloodstream, as compared with 5 to 10 percent of lead ingested from sources such as drinking water. [13]

Asbestos is another highly toxic substance found in our air. Because of its fire-retardant properties, asbestos was used for many years in a variety of building materials—from floor tiles and pipe coverings to insulation and siding. When these materials become worn or brittle, they release asbestos fibers into the air. Exposure to these particles has been shown to increase a person's risk of developing a rare form of lung cancer, mesothelioma, by anywhere from 5 to 20 times. The risk is particularly high when exposure to asbestos is coupled with smoking.

Ozone, Photochemical Air Pollution, and Smog

Smog is one of the most visible forms of air pollution. While sometimes caused by sulfur dioxide, the smog that today affects residents of Los Angeles and many other major industrialized cities is caused by **photochemical reactions**. Light energy from the sun acts upon airborne hydrocarbons and nitrogen oxides to produce a variety of new compounds. One of the most important of these is ozone.

Photochemical smog occurs in areas with poor air circulation, such as the Los Angeles valley, and it is increased by sunny weather and low humidity. A layer of cool ocean air may slip in under the normally warm, stable air above the city. Levels of photochemical air pollution rise with morning and evening rush hours. Motor-vehicle emissions rise through the cool air but cannot penetrate the warm layers, which act like a lid.

The photochemical smog that plagues many urban areas today is a complex brew of airborne pollutants. Among these are volatile organic compounds (VOCs), carbon monoxide, nitrogen

Did You Know That . . .

Up to 80 percent of the sulfate from sulfur dioxide that falls in the northeastern United States as acid rain originates in the Midwest.

Photochemical reaction(s): A chemical reaction caused by the effects of light on one or more chemicals; photochemical reactions play a significant role in the formation of smog in many urban areas.

oxides, sulfur oxides, particulates, and ozone. [14] The major source of smog-producing emissions is automobile exhaust, which contains high levels of hydrocarbons, carbon monoxide, and nitrogen oxides. However, other contributing sources include bakeries, dry-cleaners, paints, wood-burning stoves, charcoal grills, electric generating plants, and a variety of industrial processes.

One of the most harmful components of smog is ozone. Whereas the ozone that occurs naturally in the upper levels of the atmosphere performs a vital function—namely screening out ultraviolet rays from the sun—ground-level ozone is poisonous. Furthermore, ground-level ozone does not rise into the upper atmosphere, where it might ultimately be useful, but rather remains near the ground until finally swept away by prevailing winds. While present, it irritates and inflames delicate membranes in respiratory passages and impairs the oxygen-absorbing ability of our lungs. Chronic exposure can cause lesions similar to the early stages of lung cancer. [15] The immediate symptoms of exposure include shortness of breath, pain when inhaling deeply, wheezing, and coughing. These symptoms are likely to be particularly severe for asthmatics, the elderly, and heart patients. However, even trained athletes are affected. Because the effects appear to be cumulative, experts now advise against exercising when smog levels are high. [16]

Nitrogen oxides are another harmful component of smog. By-products of combustion of fossil fuels, nitrogen oxides play a role in the natural nitrogen cycle. However, there is evidence that nitrogen oxides as a component of smog cause lung tissue damage and lead to respiratory infection, flu, and the like. It is now estimated that the quantity of nitrogen oxides and sulfur oxides discharged into the atmosphere in this country annually weighs approximately 160,000 tons. This is the equivalent of tossing 4,000 loaded freight cars full of these chemicals into the air. [17]

Chlorofluorocarbons and the Ozone Layer

In the winter of 1987–88, scientists studying the Arctic made a chilling discovery. As with the Antarctic ozone layer, something was destroying the ozone layer above the Arctic. After intensive debate, scientists now agree that the culprit is the class of chemicals called chlorofluorocarbons. Inexpensive, easy to produce, and chemically inert at ground level, CFCs are used worldwide for a variety of industrial purposes. They are used as cleaning solvents for computer circuit boards and medical equipment, as refrigerants, as fire extinguishers, and as foaming agents in insulation and cushioning. [18]

(continued on p. 52)

Why No One's Safe

If you drive over the mountains into the Los Angeles basin on a hot summer day, the first thing you see is smog. The air is visible, palpable, a yellowish brown haze. It makes your eyes sting, and visitors notice coughs, sore throats and tightness in their chests—symptoms that whatever's in that air isn't good for them.

It might surprise those newcomers that many long-time residents don't notice the smog. They get used to the haze's effects. Studies have shown that long-term residents no longer recognize sore throats and eyes, though their physiological reaction to smog is the same as the non-native's. It's not unusual to hear a Los Angeleno say, "I'm immune to smog. It never affects me."

But air pollution does affect at least half the region's residents. Asthmatics, the elderly and people with heart and lung diseases or immunological problems are at risk on smoggy days. So are the two most active members of society, children and athletes.

With their developing lungs, children are perhaps the most vulnerable: One study showed that children raised in Southern California have 10% to 15% less lung function (the ability to take a deep breath) than children who grow up in less polluted air. They are also more vulnerable to pneumonia, flus and viral infections, according to Gladys Meade of the American Lung Association of California. They may be at greater risk for respiratory diseases throughout their lives.

Active children pump extra doses of smoggy air into their lungs all day long. For the same reason, smog also threatens athletes. Even at ozone levels as low as .12 parts per million (the federal standard), healthy young athletes sometimes feel headaches, shortness of breath and wheezing in endurance tests. At .20 p.p.m. of ozone, breathing becomes difficult. For most athletes, that's when performance begins to suffer.

"If you ride in the smog for more than an hour, it's painful to the lungs," says cyclist Ron Skarin. He doesn't worry about it, though, because he says studies have shown that the symptoms disappear with rest.

But recent research shows that the consequences of ozone may be permanent—and that the effects start at levels lower than the EPA standard. Robert Phalen of the Air Pollution Health Effects laboratory at the University of California at Irvine says ozone kills cells throughout the lung and loosens the junctions between cells, making the lung more vulnerable to tiny particles of pollution—and to viruses. Each time there is damage from pollutants, colds and flus, the lung repairs itself, but imperfectly. The result, says Phalen, is a sort of premature aging of the lungs. "What's more," he continues, "there may be an increased risk of lung cancer, especially for people who smoke."

Air pollution already constricts the active lifestyles of many Southern Californians, Meade says. Asthmatics have formed "Better Breathers Clubs" to walk in air-conditioned malls, where there's less ozone. Athletes must adjust their workout times to the least smoggy times in their part of the region. High school coaches have to juggle practice and game times: In San Bernardino county, where smog levels are highest at 4 p.m., games are often played in the evening or early on Saturday mornings when smog levels are lowest.

"When smog levels are high now, the Lung Association hears about headaches, dry throats, tightness of chest, a general feeling of lassitude," Meade says. "I think with clean air, people will enjoy being outside more. They'll spend time more actively, and consequently, will feel better too. Clean air will give many people an increased sense of well-being."

Source: J. E. Basu, *American Health* (September 1989), p. 64.

FIGURE 3.4

CFCs and the Ozone Layer: Measurements from the 1987 Antarctic Flights

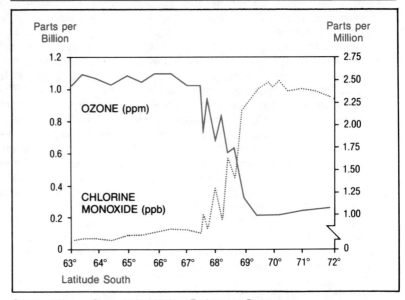

Source: *Action on Ozone,* United Nations Environment Programme.

Measurements from the 1987 Antarctic flights showed that as the scientists traveled south, levels of chlorine monoxide (a basic component of CFCs) increased and ozone levels fell.

The same chemical stability of CFCs that makes them so useful also allows them to rise up through the ozone shield into the stratosphere. Once they rise through the protective ozone shield, the CFCs are bombarded by ultraviolet radiation, which breaks them down to their basic components – chlorine, fluorine, and carbon. It is the chlorine from CFCs that is of particular concern; the chlorine atoms created by their breakdown in the upper atmosphere destroy ozone (O_3) by catalyzing its conversion to oxygen (O_2). The process is a highly efficient one, and it is estimated that every chlorine atom ultimately destroys many thousands of ozone molecules. Primarily because of the buildup of CFCs, it is estimated that the level of ozone-destroying chlorine in the upper atmosphere is now 4 to 5 times higher than normal and increasing at a rate of approximately 5 percent per year. [19]

(continued on p. 54)

What You Can Do to Save the Ozone Layer

When a health issue involves the health of the planet, people often feel that there's little they can do to change the course of events. The depletion of the earth's protective ozone layer is one of these mega-issues. While most of the measures needed to safeguard the ozone layer involve nations and industries, there are significant steps you can take—as an individual consumer and as a member of a society.

There's good and bad ozone, depending on where it is, though both are chemically identical—a gas formed when three atoms of oxygen, rather than the normal two, bind together. The ozone found at ground level, a by-product of car and factory pollution, is one of the most dangerous components of smog. But in the earth's stratosphere, about 10 to 25 miles above us, ozone functions as a natural screen against the sun's most damaging ultraviolet (UV) rays. Unfortunately, the ozone that pollutes our air cannot reach the stratosphere's ozone layer.

What CFCs do

The stratospheric ozone layer is being destroyed in large part by manmade compounds called chlorofluorocarbons, or CFCs. These versatile chemicals, in liquid or gaseous form, have helped shape modern society. CFCs are used as coolants in our homes, cars, and refrigerators; as foaming agents in foam insulation, mattresses, and food packaging; and as solvents that remove impurities from computer microchips and electronic equipment. The same properties that make CFCs efficient and safe for so many industrial uses also make them destructive for the environment. Their great stability ensures that when they are released into the air (during manufacturing, from leaky cooling systems, or upon disposal) CFCs eventually rise intact to the stratosphere, where radiation breaks them down into component atoms. One of these atoms, chlorine, has a devastating effect on ozone. Other compounds called halons, used in some fire extinguishers, are even more destructive of ozone.

Scientists predict that by allowing more UV radiation to reach the earth, the depletion of the ozone layer will lead to an increase in the number of cases of skin cancer (especially melanoma) and cataracts. In addition, they postulate that the increased UV radiation may damage crops, kill plankton that serve as a food source for marine life, and even have adverse effects on the human immune system. CFCs may also trap heat in the atmosphere and thus contribute to the global warming trend (greenhouse effect).

For all these reasons, an international agreement in Montreal in 1987 called for phasing out CFC and halon production, and [in May 1989] in Helsinki these nations agreed to accelerate the timetable. Recent reports by NASA that the ozone layer is being depleted even more rapidly than was previously projected, and the discovery of vast holes in the layer over Antarctica and the Arctic, have prompted scientists and environmental groups to call for a complete and rapid phase-out of CFCs. But even if we stopped using CFCs tomorrow, the damage to the ozone layer will continue, since those CFCs already released in the air will still be making their way to the stratosphere a decade from now and destroying ozone for up to a century.

Substitutes have already been found for certain uses of CFCs. For instance, the EPA banned the use of CFCs as propellants in most, but not all, aerosol sprays in 1978. CFCs can be modified so that they do much less damage to the ozone layer, or so that they break down quickly in the lower atmosphere. Industries are also seeking ways to recycle the chemicals so that they aren't released into the air. Du Pont, the world's largest manufacturer of CFCs, [in 1988] announced that it would phase out production by the end of the century.

Seven steps

The U.S. remains the leading producer and consumer of CFCs. By following these steps, you can help reduce the American contribution to the destruction of the ozone layer:

• Have your car's air conditioner carefully serviced. *Auto air conditioners are the single largest source of CFC emissions in the U.S.* Don't simply refill your leaky air conditioner; if you don't have the leak fixed, the CFCs you add will end up in the air. Go to a service station equipped to recycle the refrigerant (this costs an additional $35 to $55); otherwise the CFCs will be vented into the atmosphere. In Los Angeles, an ordinance requiring service stations to recycle CFCs [was] to go into effect by January 1, 1990; it [also banned] the sale of small cans of refrigerant, which allow people to "top off" their car air conditioners instead of repairing leaks. Car air conditioners using less-harmful refrigerants are expected to be available in the mid-1990s. (Home air conditioners contain coolants that are far less ozone-depleting.)

• Avoid products made of plastic foam (polystyrene), such as fast-food containers, egg cartons, Styrofoam cups, and foam trays for meats. Although many of these products are now made from less-damaging compounds, you can't tell which are which, so limit your use of them.

• Don't use foam plastic insulation in your home, unless it is made with ozone-safe agents. Or use fiberglass, gypsum, fiberboard, or cellulose insulation.

• Don't buy a halon fire extinguisher for home use.

• Check labels on aerosol cans. VCR-head cleaners, boat horns, spray confetti, photo-negative cleaners, and drain plungers are still allowed to contain the most dangerous CFCs. Many cans say if they contain CFCs, but such labeling isn't required.

• When buying a refrigerator, choose an energy-efficient model: it may contain as little as half the CFCs. Thus when the fridge wears out and you dump it, less CFCs will be released. All refrigerators sold in the U.S. contain CFCs. To keep your fridge in the best working order, clean the coils regularly; that way it may last until CFC-free models are developed, or at least until recycling programs for CFCs are available.

• If you feel strongly, write to your Senator and Representative and to President Bush, urging them to protect the ozone layer by tightening regulations on CFCs and halons, speeding up their elimination, mandating warning labels on products containing them, and pressing other nations to take such steps.

Substitutes for CFCs may add to the cost of many products, be less efficient, and have other drawbacks, at least at first. This may be hard to accept, especially since CFC emissions are invisible, and most of the damage they cause may not become evident for decades. But the steps we take now to protect the ozone layer will benefit our grandchildren.

Source: *University of California Berkeley Wellness Letter,* Vol. 6, No. 1, October 1989, p. 7.

As noted earlier, one of the functions of the ozone layer is to absorb ultraviolet radiation from the sun. As the ozone layer is depleted, an increasing proportion of the sun's ultraviolet radiation reaches the Earth's surface. The primary health risk associated with this development is a greatly increased risk of a variety of cancers, particularly skin cancers. The Environmental Protection Agency has estimated that ozone depletion will lead to an additional 31,000 to 126,000 cases of melanoma, the most dangerous form of skin cancer, among U.S. whites born before 1975, and an additional 7,000 to 30,000 deaths. [20] Other health risks

Table 3.1 Common Outdoor Air Pollution Problems

Pollutant	Number of U.S. Counties Currently Exceeding Federal Health Standard	Population Potentially Exposed	Trend	Comments
Ozone	341	126,809,800	probably on increase	worst urban air problem
Carbon Monoxide	125	89,009,900	decreasing now	expected to worsen in 1990's
Particulate Matter	122	54,564,300	probably increasing	pollution control program stalled since 1982
Sulfur Dioxide	50	14,109,400	decreasing	short-term protection inadequate
Nitrogen Dioxide	4	12,138,100	increasing	fastest growing pollutant
Lead	N/A	N/A	has decreased dramatically	EPA should ban lead in gas

N/A = not available

Source: *Facts About Air Pollution and Your Health,* American Lung Association, 1988, p. 4.

associated with the depletion of the ozone layer include an increased incidence of cataracts and the possible depression of the immune system. [21]

Chlorofluorocarbons have another potentially harmful property: they contribute to the greenhouse effect. For example, it is estimated that one molecule of CFC-11 or CFC-12, 2 types of chlorofluorocarbons, can trap as much heat as 10,000 molecules of carbon dioxide. Although CFCs are not thought to have a direct effect on human health, their roles in the depletion of the ozone layer and in the expansion of the greenhouse effect make it important to limit their use.

Limited attempts to do this are now under way. The first of these occurred in the late 1970s when the EPA banned their use as aerosol propellants. However, the potential magnitude of the impact of CFCs on the ozone layer did not become apparent until the first published reports of a "hole" in the ozone layer over Antarctica appeared in 1984–85. These reports and the many similar findings that followed, coupled with the fact that CFCs are used worldwide, have prompted international action. The

Montreal Protocol on substances that deplete the ozone layer was established on September 16, 1987, and has since been signed by 35 countries. In May 1989, the signatory countries informally pledged to ban CFCs altogether by the year 2000. Nonetheless, CFC production continues and seems unlikely to end until and unless the problems associated with their use become even more urgent, or safe and inexpensive substitutes are developed.

INDOOR POLLUTION

If you think that you can come in from the elements outside and be safe indoors, you should think again. Many of the atmospheric pollutants seep into our homes and offices, of course, but once there, they are joined by a host of other substances. In recent years, awareness of what lurks in flooring and carpets (formaldehyde to make us dizzy), air conditioning (mold and bacteria), closets (dry-cleaning chemicals and those from synthetic fibers), showers (chloroform in water that went through sewage-treatment plants), and even the very foundation of our buildings (radon to raise the risk of cancer) has generated new terms such as "sick building syndrome" and new approaches to wellness such as **clinical ecology.** Because it is often difficult to link a given set of symptoms to a single, specific environmental cause, many claims of sickness linked to indoor air pollution are met by skepticism among the medical establishment, the business community, and even the general public. But since an estimated 11,000 deaths yearly and acquired and irreversible allergies can be traced to the effects of indoor pollution, we should be alert for ways to avoid specific problems. We are not talking of the substances—dust, pollen, animal fur—that affect a sensitive allergic person; we restrict ourselves here to the ways the environment—and what human activity does to it—is hazardous to the health of all of us.

Ironically, a large part of the problem originated with the drive to save energy in the 1970s. One result was "tighter" houses, which keep in not only heat but, unfortunately, pollutants. Of course, fumes from burning wood were irritants to earlier civilizations, including the teepee dwellers in America. Today, however, we are exposed to an ever-increasing number of man-made chemicals; the American Academy of Environmental Medicine examined global data and found 60,000 chemical combinations are introduced each month. [22] Some of them are making us sick. The EPA has identified over 3,000 substances in indoor

Clinical ecology: A subfield of ecology concerned with the clinical effects of the environment on health.

FIGURE 3.5
Sources of Indoor Air Pollution

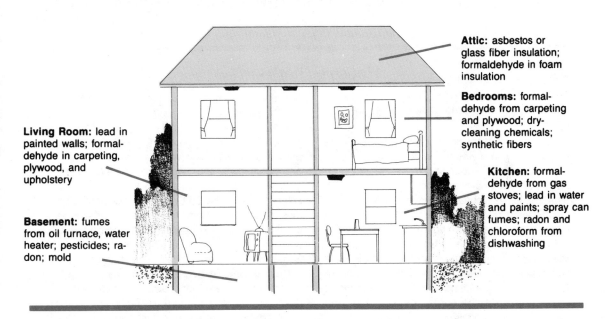

Attic: asbestos or glass fiber insulation; formaldehyde in foam insulation

Bedrooms: formaldehyde from carpeting and plywood; dry-cleaning chemicals; synthetic fibers

Living Room: lead in painted walls; formaldehyde in carpeting, plywood, and upholstery

Kitchen: formaldehyde from gas stoves; lead in water and paints; spray can fumes; radon and chloroform from dishwashing

Basement: fumes from oil furnace, water heater; pesticides; radon; mold

Sources of indoor pollution may be found in every room of a house.

air that are potential health problems. Interestingly, the EPA's own Washington, D.C., headquarters was found to be one of the 20 percent of all new commercial buildings that have unhealthy air.

Leading Indoor Pollutants

Asbestos, once hailed as a life-saving, fire-resistant, insulating material, has been properly getting bad press in recent years. Its tiny fibers can get into lungs, remaining to cause scarring of lung tissue, coronary problems, and lung and other cancers. When it remains intact, it generally does little harm. However, its tendency to flake off and penetrate the air or duct systems is driving school systems and many others to go to the costly trouble of removing it—work that must be performed by certified contractors. Virtually all uses have been banned.

Formaldehyde—a component of the binding agents used in

Asbestos: A naturally occurring fibrous mineral that is widely used in insulating and fireproofing materials; exposure to asbestos has been linked to lung cancer.

Formaldehyde: A colorless, pungent gas that is both suffocating and poisonous in high dosages; formaldehyde is a component of a variety of resins and plastics that are widely used as building materials.

a variety of construction materials, adhesives, and furnishings—releases a gas that can produce a variety of reactions: respiratory and skin irritations, nausea, dizziness. It may also be a depressant of the central nervous system and a source of cancer. Installation of new carpeting treated with it may cause office

(continued on p. 60)

Houses That Hurt

Thad Godish had barely entered the house before he said, "Ann, I know what's wrong with you."

For Ann Hardacre of Anderson, Ind., a terrifying, debilitating mystery was at last at an end. She had been ill for four long years. Her stomach hurt, she had severe headaches, she ached all over, she felt as if she had a never-ending case of the flu—and doctor after doctor had been baffled. "I was like a drowning person," she recalls.

But the trained nose of Dr. Godish, director of the indoor air quality research lab at Ball State University, had detected the telltale fumes of formaldehyde emanating from the pressed-wood products used in the home's construction. Ann Hardacre's *house* was making her ill.

Though her symptoms were more extreme than most, millions of people are now believed to suffer to some extent from what is called "sick house syndrome." In older houses it can be caused by mold, bacteria, antiquated plumbing that sheds lead into the drinking water, or aged heating systems that produce too much carbon monoxide and other harmful gases. Houses of all ages may, depending on their location, be subject to contamination by radon, a naturally occurring radioactive gas emanating from the soil, whose byproducts can cause lung cancer. But more and more often, the sick house is equated with the modern house.

It incorporates new materials and furnishings that exude dangerous chemicals, for one thing. And building standards aimed at energy efficiency have made it difficult for homes to exhale them: Many of today's homes are semisealed boxes that don't "breathe" well, leaving noxious fumes confined inside. "Energy-efficient means

pollution-efficient, too," says one environmental health specialist.

Today's houses are full of chemicals—carcinogens, allergic agents, irritants—that can make people sick. Formaldehyde, a simple but dangerous chemical that has been linked to cancer and other health effects, is ubiquitous. Particleboard and plywood, common building materials today, are held together by adhesives containing it. It's also present in furniture fabric, permanent-press clothing, paints, cosmetics, detergents, even paper towels.

Hazard lurks in every room. Today's carpets are often treated with powerful chemicals to resist stains, and modern sealants and glues often contain substances harmful to some people. Scented products such as mothballs are loaded with toxic irritants. Closets full of dry-cleaned clothes exhale tetrachloroethylene, a cancer-causing agent, and another one, chloroform, may vaporize out of the water supply when someone turns on the shower. Even low-level electromagnetic radiation—emitted by local power lines but also by microwave ovens, home computers, and even portable phones and electric blankets—is suspect.

The sick-house syndrome is now getting a lot more attention. Earon Davis, publisher of Ecological Illness Law Report in Wilmette, Ill., says lawsuits against makers of building materials, household pesticides and consumer products that cause sickness are gaining credibility. "There are more victims," he says, "and more physicians willing to testify."

It wasn't always so. Back in the 1950s, Pheron Randolph, now 83 and still practicing medicine, was ridiculed when he told a national meeting of allergists that the hydrocarbons emitted by gas-fired kitchen stoves and ranges were responsible for headaches, fatigue, bronchitis, asthma, arthritis and depression in many of his patients.

"The other allergists thought this was hilariously funny and guffawed all over the place," recalls Dr. Randolph. There are far fewer scoffers now. Dr. Randolph says he has improved the health of some 4,000 patients by ordering gas stoves out of their homes.

Though most people don't have any noticeable or immediate reaction to harmful substances in the home atmosphere, a sizable minority may suffer in silence from itchy eyes, runny noses, sinus or lung congestion, constant fatigue or depression without realizing why. William Rea, head of the Environmental Health Center in Dallas and a former president of the American Academy of Environmental Medicine, estimates that 20% of the U.S. population suffers from chemical sensitivities.

Some people can become very ill indeed. Exposure to harmful fumes in the home may trigger full-blown, broad-scale allergic responses in people who weren't noticeably allergic before, forcing them to live restricted lives. That's what happened to Ann Hardacre.

When she and her husband heard that their house was the cause of her symptoms, they purged it. Particleboard floors loaded with formaldehyde were ripped up, and plywood, paneling and other pressed-wood products were removed. Glass-fiber furnace pipes, which were giving off fumes, were replaced. Today Mrs. Hardacre, now 57, has no major problems with the house, but she remains highly allergic to a host of substances.

She can wear clothing made only from natural fibers, and even at that she must wash new garments in baking soda before she wears them. She drinks mineral water bottled only in glass because she has become allergic to soft plastic. When the newspaper arrives in the morning, she puts it in the microwave oven for a minute or so to dry the ink. Ironically, her home—"my oasis," she calls it—is now her best refuge from the broad range of pollutants and chemicals to which she has grown so sensitive.

Today's tightly built, energy-efficient houses not only confine more chemical fumes but also worsen the radon problem, which is widespread; The Environmental Protection Agency found that 25% of the homes it tested in 17 states contained radon in excess of EPA standards. The worst areas: Minnesota, North Dakota and along the geological formation called the Reading Prong, which cuts through parts of New York, New Jersey and Pennsylvania.

Homeowners usually can bring radon readings to safe levels by sealing off basements and installing ventilation devices that will move the gas from beneath the house and out into the open air, where it disperses. Chemicals that are literally built into the structure of the whole house, however, are harder to deal with. Like Mrs. Hardacre, highly sensitive people often have no choice but to rip out the offending materials, a costly process, or start from scratch in a new home.

Healthier homes are now being designed. Clint Good, a Washington, D.C., architect and author of a book called "Healthful Houses," uses only natural and nontoxic products in home construction. He favors solid-wood floors and cabinetry, for example, and marble or tile for kitchen and bathroom surfaces. Instead of standard tile adhesive, he opts for cement-based mortar, and he recommends aluminum-foil insulation.

Similarly, some architects are recommending electric and solar energy over oil and natural gas. Others design new homes with air-to-air exchangers that expel warm, stale air and transfer the heat to fresh air coming in, allowing the interior to "breathe." And an array of nontoxic paints, sealers, cleansers, adhesives and other materials is hitting the market, too. All this can push up the cost of a house by a goodly sum—but if the less-toxic environment is medically required, Mr. Good notes, the extra costs can be deducted at income-tax time.

Source: D. Goldberg, *Wall Street Journal* (19 May 1989), p. R29.

Prior to August 1990, when the EPA banned its use in paints intended for interior use, mercury was commonly used in latex paint to help retard the growth of mildew.

Nitrogen dioxide (NO₂): A reddish-brown, highly poisonous gas present in the exhaust of internal-combustion engines that is a major air pollutant in many urban areas.

Secondhand smoke: Tobacco smoke that is inhaled by nonsmokers.

Lead: A heavy, comparatively soft metal that is easy to work and most commonly found in nature combined as a sulfide; lead is poisonous when absorbed by the body.

Radon: A naturally occurring, radioactive, gaseous element that is a product of radium decay; high radon levels that build up in enclosed areas are a potential health hazard.

workers to be ill for months. Formaldehyde is also produced in some combustion processes; gas stoves are an overlooked source.

Carbon monoxide, **nitrogen dioxide**, and sulfur dioxide are as serious—perhaps more so—indoors as out. The major sources of these pollutants are kerosene heaters, furnaces, and car exhaust entering homes from attached garages. We now know that exposure to **secondhand smoke** exposes nonsmokers to nicotine, formaldehyde, arsenic, carbon monoxide, and much else. Inhaling large quantities of these chemicals can result in breathing problems, eye irritation, nausea, and increased risk of heart disease and cancer.

Government regulations have led to the removal of **lead** from paints. However, many older homes still contain surfaces covered with lead paint. These pose the greatest potential danger to children, who are likely to ingest paint chips. And adults and children alike are exposed to lead used in older plumbing systems.

Radon is a colorless, odorless, radioactive gas that originates with uranium in the soil beneath buildings and has been linked to lung cancer. Although some areas are known for higher than usual quantities, its presence is a highly localized situation, with enormous variance from neighbor to neighbor. Levels do not have to be very high to emit radiation equal to what you would receive from hundreds of chest X rays in a year, but there are tests for its detection and several approaches, especially ventilation systems, that *can* effectively reduce it.

Radon is a natural pollutant, but most pollutants are not. Very often, our problems originate with materials and processes that we have devised to save labor or time or to make our personal and working worlds more productive, convenient, or comfortable. The ecology-minded *Amicus Journal* has called environmental illness the "ultimate 20th century illness, affecting 15 percent of the population." [23] Some advances have resulted in increased life spans and improved health. Others have made life easier, and still others are unnecessary or just plain silly. Room deodorizers and moth repellents, for example, may contain paradichlorobenzene, which researchers say has caused cancer in rats. So the combatants in the war against pollution are not only industries, environmentalists, and our federal, state, and local governments; Los Angeles would still not meet federal air-quality standards if every single industry completely eliminated its emissions. As one observer put it, the *real* regulatory targets "have mushroomed from 200,000 large or industrial sources to 240 million small ones: people." [24]

(continued on p. 62)

Home Indoor Air Quality Checklist

The average American is indoors nearly 90 percent of the time, and more than half of this is spent in the home.

This checklist is a guide to determine the general status of indoor air quality in the home.
Answer "yes" or "no" to each of the following questions.

Sources Of Indoor Contaminants

____ ■ Do you have any unvented gas appliances?

____ ■ Do any household members smoke? (Add one "yes" for each.)

____ ■ Do any furry pets live indoors? (Add one "yes" for each pet.)

____ ■ Do you have any house plants?

____ ■ Are insecticides or pesticides used indoors?

____ ■ How many cars are parked in an attached enclosed garage? (Add one "yes" for each car.)

____ ■ Are any of the following hobbies conducted indoors: woodworking, jewelry making, pottery or model building?

____ ■ Do you use pressurized aerosol canisters?

____ ■ Is part of your living area below ground?

____ ■ Is your house insulated with ureaformaldehyde or asbestos?

____ ■ Are heating vents corroded or rusted?

____ ■ Do burner flames on gas-heating or cooking appliances appear yellow instead of blue?

Strength of Indoor Contaminants

____ ■ Are there unusual and noticeable odors?

____ ■ Is the humidity level unusually high or is moisture noticeable on windows or other surfaces?

____ ■ Does the air seem stale?

____ ■ Are any of the following symptoms noticeable among residents: headaches, itchy or watery eyes, nose or throat infection or dryness, dizziness, nausea, colds, sinus problems?

____ ■ Is the house temperature unusually warm or cold?

____ ■ Is there a noticeable lack of air movement?

____ ■ Is dust on furniture noticeable?

____ ■ Is dust or dirt staining walls, ceilings, furniture or draperies?

____ ■ Have you weatherized your home recently?

High-Risk Household Members

____ ■ Are any family members less than four or more than 60 years old?

____ ■ Is anyone normally confined to the house more than 12 hours per day?

____ ■ Does anyone suffer from asthma or bronchitis, allergies, heart problems or hypersensitivity pneumonitis?

Give yourself one point for each "yes" answer to the preceding questions.

____ *TOTAL "YES" ANSWERS*

In general, more than ten "yes" answers may indicate poor indoor air quality.

Implementing some of the control measures listed below will improve indoor air quality. A severe problem associated with any one of these questions, however, may require immediate corrective action.

You can also call your local Lung Association or health agency to request more information or to ask about a professional evaluation of your home's air quality.

Indoor Air Quality Control Measures

■ Ask smokers to confine smoking to one room in house or go outdoors.
■ Use nonaerosol products.
■ Install exhaust fans in bathrooms.
■ Fit gas ranges with hood fans that exhaust outside. Use the fan or open a window while cooking.
■ Use a portable air cleaner, or install a medium/high efficiency media air filter or electronic air cleaner in forced-air heating/cooling system.
■ Install activated charcoal, aluminum or other type of gaseous air cleaner in forced-air heating/cooling system.
■ Have furnace, gas water heater and clothes dryer inspected regularly.
■ Continually operate the forced-air fan.
■ Leave doors between rooms open most of the time.
■ Leave some windows partially opened.
■ Install outdoor air intake to return-air ductwork of forced-air system.
■ Clean air conditioners, air ducts, humidifiers, heat exchangers and microwave ovens regularly.

Source: American Lung Association, 1986.

CONSCIOUSNESS, WELLNESS LEVELS, AND THE RAISING OF THEM

When we are told that in a century, the Earth's average temperature will rise a few degrees, we may not get excited. As any newspaper reporter knows, facts have to have relevance to the reader to have any impact as news. But as we have seen, this temperature change is symptomatic of more profound changes that we *should* clamor about. A man-made imbalance in our air could eventually change our entire history. Or as one scenario had it, ice caps would melt, oceans would swell, coastal areas would flood, and the Miami Dolphins would retreat to Calgary, Canada. [25]

The federal Clean Air Act, passed in 1970 and amended in 1977, signaled a major change in our consciousness of the importance of air quality. It established strict air-quality standards based primarily on *health* rather than economic considerations. The Clean Air Act empowered the Environmental Protection Agency (EPA), also established in 1970, to set limits on several major air pollutants, including sulfur oxides and nitrogen oxides, and it mandated reduction of automobile and factory emissions. The EPA has spent much of its short existence in a tug-of-war

FIGURE 3.6
Where It Hurts: Health Effects of Pollution

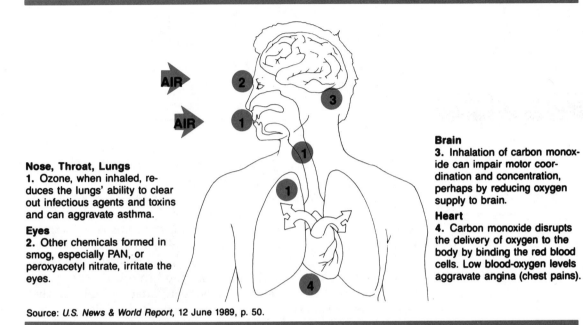

Nose, Throat, Lungs
1. Ozone, when inhaled, reduces the lungs' ability to clear out infectious agents and toxins and can aggravate asthma.

Eyes
2. Other chemicals formed in smog, especially PAN, or peroxyacetyl nitrate, irritate the eyes.

Brain
3. Inhalation of carbon monoxide can impair motor coordination and concentration, perhaps by reducing oxygen supply to brain.

Heart
4. Carbon monoxide disrupts the delivery of oxygen to the body by binding the red blood cells. Low blood-oxygen levels aggravate angina (chest pains).

Source: *U.S. News & World Report*, 12 June 1989, p. 50.

Pollutants and toxic chemicals in the air can cause many health problems.

between the liberalism of the 1970s and the conservatism that took over in the 1980s. The automobile industry was told to reduce its emissions by 90 percent. Battle lines were drawn: industrialists claimed that the price of compliance was too high; environmentalists countered that increased costs would be balanced by a reduction in pollution-related illness and deaths (one estimate puts medical bills avoided by pollution control at $40 billion per year). [26] Headlines screamed, tempers flared—and yet today's new cars produce an average of only 4 percent as much pollution as 1970 models. [27] But we still have a long way to go. When one of the largest factories in the United States pumped 6 million pounds of toxic chemicals into the surrounding sky in the course of a year, the company's vice president stated, "We do put up big numbers, but every one of those pounds going into the air is in compliance with the law." [28] Clearly, there is still room for improvement in the battle against air pollution.

4

At Risk:
Good Water

I T SEEMS THAT 1989 was the year of the oil spills. The Exxon *Valdez* dumped 11 million gallons of oil into Alaska's Prince William Sound on March 24. Then just 3 months later, on June 24, within a 12-hour period, oil first spilled into the waters of Rhode Island, then Texas, and then Delaware. Coast Guard data show that spills are frequent events. From 1984 through 1988, there were 15,260 reported incidents that dumped some 32 million gallons of oil into U.S. waters. [1] Oil spills, no matter where they happen, affect us all, for the Earth's water supply is a single, interconnected whole.

> On Earth is only one body of water, which is constantly travel-ing from one river to one lake to one ocean. Water frozen today into glaciers and icebergs is tomorrow bathing tropical shores. Unchanged, perennial, the water of the ocean runs along the coastlines of deserts, paradise islands, rocky cliffs, flat marshes, and a hundred varied countries. These hundred nations differ by their people, their degree of development, their religious beliefs, their political regimes, and their administrative struc-tures. But to all, the sea is a bonus, soothing climates, washing beaches, feeding animals and people, and connecting nations. [2]

The importance of the oceans is matched by that of the inland waterways that supply an essential resource–drinking water.

SUPPLY AND DEMAND

Because the Earth's water supply is continually replenished through the workings of the **hydrologic cycle**, water is often looked upon as a renewable resource. And, after all, doesn't water

Hydrologic cycle: The natural sequence through which water circulates in the biosphere; surface water passes into the Earth's atmosphere in the form of water vapor (via the process of evaporation), falls from the atmosphere in the form of rain, snow, or other precip-itation, and ultimately returns to the atmosphere through evaporation.

64

FIGURE 4.1
Our Water Supply: Where It Comes From

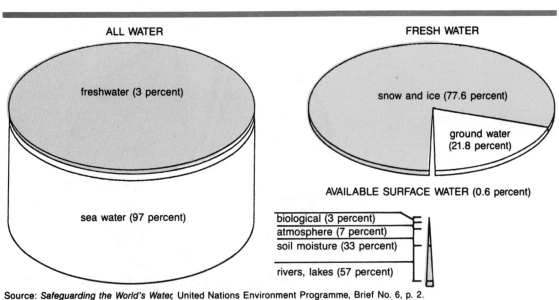

ALL WATER

freshwater (3 percent)

sea water (97 percent)

FRESH WATER

snow and ice (77.6 percent)

ground water
(21.8 percent)

AVAILABLE SURFACE WATER (0.6 percent)

biological (3 percent)
atmosphere (7 percent)
soil moisture (33 percent)

rivers, lakes (57 percent)

Source: *Safeguarding the World's Water,* United Nations Environment Programme, Brief No. 6, p. 2.

The total volume of water on Earth is about 1,400 million cubic kilometers, of which 97 percent is sea water. Of the remaining freshwater supply, less than 1 percent is available for human use.

cover most of the surface of the planet? Well, the fact is that less than 1 percent of Earth's water is available for us to drink. To understand this, imagine that the total planetary water supply is 38 liters (10 gallons). After we take out the ocean water that is too salty for drinking, for growing crops, and for most industrial purposes, about 1.1 liters (4.5 cups) remain. Of this, about 0.83 liter (3.5 cups) lies too far under the Earth's surface or is tied up in glaciers, in ice caps, in the atmosphere, and in the soil as "bound water," unavailable for use by plants or for extraction by wells. This leaves only about 0.27 liter (1 cup). When we take out the water that is polluted, relatively inaccessible, or too expensive to get to, the remaining supply of usable fresh water is only about 0.001 liter (or 10 drops). [3]

As if that isn't problematic enough: the 1 percent of the available water is unequally distributed. New York City's needs are too great to be met by only the Hudson River, so it taps into its

FIGURE 4.2
Our Water Supply: Where It Goes

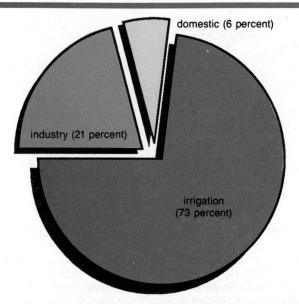

domestic (6 percent)

industry (21 percent)

irrigation
(73 percent)

Source: *Safeguarding the World's Water*, United Nations Environment Programme, Brief No. 6,
p. 3.

Fresh water is primarily used for agriculture, industry, and domestic purposes. Irrigation, which accounts for the bulk of agricultural use, is very wasteful. Often more than 70 percent of the water used for irrigation never reaches the crops.

neighbors' Upper Delaware River for more. This in turn causes Philadelphia to run short, so Philadelphia looks to the Susquehanna River. Water from the Colorado River is piped to quench the great thirst of Los Angeles. Other water-short states are also looking for pipeline bailouts. [4] Periods of drought— bound to increase with global warming—affect every part of the planet. If 1989 was the year of spills, 1988 was a record year of dry weather for the United States, a year that witnessed the destruction of grains and soybeans that would have fed the hungry around the world, and the backing up of saltwater into drinking water supplies as streams and reservoirs became lower. The resulting smaller ponds and lakes, with less fresh water and higher water temperatures and concentrations of toxic substances, became filled with dead and dying fish and waterfowl.

These shortages have presented some bizarre entrepre-neurial efforts. A Paradise, California, company has proposed a $120-billion scheme for delivering water to the Southwest from the water-rich Canadian provinces of British Columbia and the Yukon and the state of Alaska. A Torrance, California, man has offered to tow a giant Antarctic iceberg to the California coast for $65 million—with delivery only 120 days from the time the order is placed. The idea excited Arabian sheiks, whose water prices were already greater than the price of oil on a per-barrel basis. [5] And, of course, the idea of **desalinization**—the process of remov-ing salt from seawater—is always brought up wherever fresh water is scarce. This is an exceedingly expensive solution: Saudi Arabia spent $15 billion in a 3-year period on the process. [6] The United States, Israel, and other nations needing agricultural irrigation must actually "mine" water, drilling into currents deep under ground. The Ogallala aquifer (a water-bearing layer of permeable rock, sand, or gravel) under the Great Plains of the United States has been drained of 25 percent of its resources. Russia's Aral Sea has been shrunk by 40 percent.

Clearly, there are not as many drops to drink as we thought. If we are not to run short of this essential resource, we need to look for ways to decrease consumption while protecting the quality of our remaining supplies.

WHAT CONSTITUTES WATER POLLUTION?

It should be noted at this point that just as there is no such thing as "pure" air, so there is no such thing in nature as "pure" water. Water (H_2O), sometimes known as the universal solvent, reacts with many other substances. All naturally occurring water con-tains contaminants—salt, organic matter from decaying vege-tation, and a variety of other substances. Some of these contaminants (essential minerals, for example) are beneficial. Others, such as asbestos and radon, are harmful if ingested in sufficient doses.

Water pollution occurs when water is contaminated by the addition of organic and industrial waste so that it fails to meet water-quality standards or cannot be used for a specific purpose. Water that is too polluted to drink may be satisfactory for industrial use. Water too polluted for swimming may not be too polluted for fishing. Water too polluted for fishing may still be suitable for boating or for generating electrical power.

Even though scientists have developed sensitive measuring

Desalinization: The removal of salt and other substances from water (usually seawater) to make it drinkable; also known as desalination.

Water pollution: The contamination of water by impurities, including decaying organic matter, chemicals, dissolved gases, and suspended solids.

*Recipe for
Pollution Soup*

To contaminating agricultural and industrial runoff discharged by rivers and streams into estuaries, add the following lethal ingredients:
- sulfuric and nitric acids from acid rain
- toxic chemicals from wind-borne pesticides
- oil spills from tankers and offshore drilling rigs
- uncounted tons of garbage (mainly nonbiodegradable plastics) dumped from oceangoing ships, fishermen, and recreational boaters
- raw human and animal sewage
- radioactive wastes
- dioxin-laced ash from ocean incinerators and illegal dump ships
- medical and surgical debris

   Mix thoroughly and run like the plague (not recommended for eating, washing, swimming, or drinking).

Source: J. Naar, *Design for a Livable Planet: How You Can Help Clean Up the Environment* (New York: HarperCollins, 1990).

instruments, determining water quality is difficult. Screening for contaminants becomes an enormously complex process when the list of potential suspects includes the estimated 63,000 chemicals used commercially, many of which are present only in trace amounts. Determining the exact form and concentration of these myriad substances and their effects on humans and other organisms is extremely difficult and expensive. Yet it is vital to our well-being. Water is a necessity for all forms of life on Earth, and the availability of an adequate supply of usable water is vital to the development of human communities.

As noted earlier, each of us is almost 70 percent water, and we require 2 to 3 quarts of water each day to meet our bodily needs. Multiply one person's needs by our exploding numbers and you begin to realize the extent of the demand for water. In the vital matter of finding and maintaining good water, we have not been doing ourselves any favors. Crowded cities (with half the population living within 50 miles of an ocean), technological advances, and, of course, plain carelessness have routinely contaminated our water supplies, sometimes turning them into a hazardous stew.

Even so, water quality in the United States is an antipollution success story. Thirty or 40 years ago, industrial wastes had turned many bodies of fresh water into corpses. In 1969 the ahoga River in Ohio even caught fire when the oil that had accumulated on it was ignited. Lake Erie was pronounced dead in 1960, but it is today alive and well. The water quality of New York's Hudson River has improved significantly, and various other areas no longer make for scary headlines and idle fishermen. These developments illustrate once again the resilience of our ecosystem. Still, the EPA has identified 700 toxic substances in U.S. water systems, and the quality of many of our drinking-water sources is constantly being threatened by continuing discharges and by increasing demand.

Chemicals in the Water

Regardless of where they are disposed of first, chemicals generally end up in the water. Pollutants in the atmosphere are washed out of the sky by the rain, chemicals discarded in landfills creep into nearby water, and agricultural chemicals run off the land into lakes and rivers. Some of these substances, such as mercury, cadmium, arsenic, and nitrates, are inorganic. Others, such as polychlorinated biphenyls (**PCBs**), oil, and **pesticides**, are organic chemicals, carbon-based compounds derived from living things. These are but a few of the unwanted substances in our water supply.

One of the most common inorganic pollutants is lead. Although not found free in nature, it has a long history of human use. It was known to the Egyptians and ancient Babylonians and used extensively by the Romans for water pipes. The word "plumbing" is, in fact, derived from the Latin name for lead, *plumbum*. Lead has a low melting point, is easily cast, and is widely used in a variety of manufacturing processes. It is a basic component of many batteries and was, until recently, also found in most paints and many brands of gasoline.

Although lead is still widely used for many manufacturing purposes, its use in plumbing, pottery, paints, and any other uses that involve the risk of human consumption or ingestion is now generally prohibited in the United States. Lead is a highly toxic substance, and all lead compounds are poisonous. Although this has long been known, it is only in relatively recent times that evidence implicating lead as a major health risk became available. In part, this is because the progress of lead poisoning is very gradual, often extending over many years. Furthermore, the early symptoms—gradual weakness, constipation, anemia—are easily overlooked or attributed to other causes. It is now thought that a number of the Roman emperors, such as Caligula, Claudius, and Nero, may have suffered from chronic lead poisoning,

Did You Know That . . .

Water runoff from Mount Fuji in Japan is said by environmental experts to be so alkaline that it can be used to develop photographic film.

PCB(s): The common abbreviation of the chemical name polychlorinated biphenyl, which applies to several mixtures of organic compounds produced by the reaction of chlorine with biphenyl; widely used as lubricants and heat-transfer fluids in electrical equipment, especially transformers, PCBs are toxic and resist decomposition.

Pesticide(s): Any chemical or substance used to destroy one or more species of pests (usually insects); while some pesticides are natural in origin, most are man-made.

Did You Know That . . .

I n spite of the fact that Congress passed the Safe Drinking Water Act nearly two decades ago, the drinking water consumed by approximately 1 in 6 Americans contains excessive amounts of lead.

which contributed to their bizarre behavior. If so, their major source of exposure to lead probably occurred when drinking a grape-juice syrup that was brewed in lead pots and then used to sweeten foods and wine. [7]

Although lead is no longer used in plumbing or paints in this country, and its use in gasoline is being phased out, it remains a substantial and significant pollutant in our water supply, affecting an estimated 1 in 6 households. [8] A lead concentration above 10 micrograms per liter is considered unsafe. However, because lead's effects are so subtle, lead contamination often goes unnoticed. Given the continued presence of lead in older plumbing systems and its continuing use in a variety of manufacturing processes where it is sometimes discharged into the air (from whence it ultimately enters the water supply), lead continues to be a significant health risk.

Another important inorganic water pollutant is mercury. A deadly poison, mercury enters the water supply from a number of sources. In the past, the most important of these was industrial pollution from chlorine-caustic soda (sodium hydroxide) plants and pulp and paper mills. Today strict laws regulate the discharge of mercury by industry. However, as a result of the burning of fossil fuels and mercury ore refining, processes that discharge mercury into the atmosphere, some mercury finds its way back to the Earth via rainfall. Minute amounts of mercury can add up to serious trouble. Some parts of the body, such as the brain, tend to retain mercury over the years, and its cumulative toxic effects on the nervous system are irreversible; vision and hearing problems can also result. Those with nutritional deficiencies (of magnesium or thiamine, for example) seem more susceptible to damage. Fetuses exposed to mercury are at high risk for mercury-contamination-related cerebral palsy.

Like lead, cadmium does not naturally occur in free form. Its presence in water results entirely from industrial processes. Cadmium, a marvelous plating agent, is used in the manufacture of many items, including paints and pesticides. In some areas, wastes from electroplating plants and cadmium-containing products buried in landfills have contaminated groundwaters, giving rise to concerns that cadmium is being released into the air as a result of burning at these dumps. Cadmium is also found in tobacco products. Its effects on humans are insidious: once cadmium is absorbed by the body, as many as 10 to 30 years may pass before it is excreted. The harmful effects of cadmium ingestion include kidney damage, pulmonary disease, and possibly high blood pressure. [9]

(continued on p. 72)

FIGURE 4.3
Sources of Water Pollution

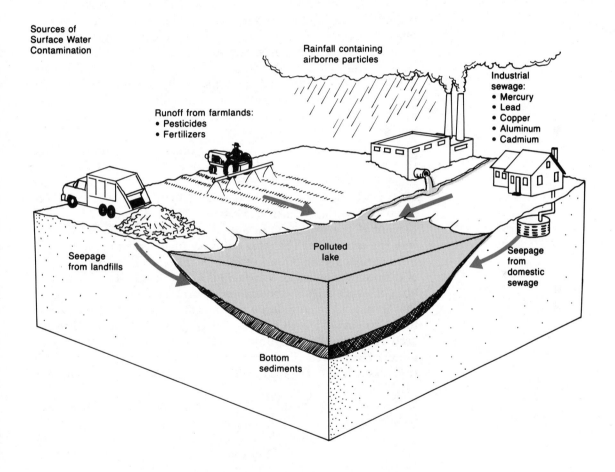

Sources of
Surface Water
Contamination

Rainfall containing
airborne particles

Industrial
sewage:
• Mercury
• Lead
• Copper
• Aluminum
• Cadmium

Runoff from farmlands:
• Pesticides
• Fertilizers

Seepage
from landfills

Polluted
lake

Seepage
from
domestic
sewage

Bottom
sediments

Source: Robert Italiano.

Chemicals can enter a lake, river, or stream from landfills that are not properly sealed, and from industrial and domestic sewage plants. Pesticides and fertilizers from farming and airborne chemicals from power plants and other industries contaminate freshwater sources through rainfall and runoff.

Other inorganic pollutants found in our water supply include copper particles and aluminum. Both are highly toxic. High levels of copper can cause debilitating diarrhea and fever as well as anemia and heart problems. Aluminum can replace the calcium in the body that is necessary to human health, and can contribute to or cause kidney and general neurological damage. It may also contribute to Alzheimer's disease.

While radon is primarily thought of as an airborne pollutant, radon in household water accounts for as many as 1,800 deaths a year. Showering, dishwashing, and laundering agitate water, which releases radon into the air. It has been estimated that waterborne radon may cause more cancer deaths than all other drinking-water pollutants combined. [10] As many as 8 million people may have undesirably high radon levels in the water they obtain from private wells or community water systems that are too small to disperse the gas.

Many of the important water pollutants are organic. One that has received much publicity in recent years is oil. Sadly, the much publicized spills of 1989 were far exceeded by the quantity of oil discharged into the Persian Gulf during the 1991 Gulf War. Even before this occurred, it was estimated that 1 tenth of 1 percent of the world's total annual oil production found its way into the ocean. [11] The total quantity involved, approximately 5 million tons a year, equals roughly 1 gram per 100 square meters of the ocean's surface. Because oil is almost completely biodegradable, it eventually evaporates or is broken down by bacteria. If this were not the case, large portions of the ocean's surface would today be covered with oil. We can be grateful that this has not occurred, but the continuing discharge of oil into the Earth's oceans has destructive effects on marine life and, insofar as it finds its way into the food chain, poses a potential risk to human health.

As with several other water pollutants, the problems posed by the highly toxic family of organic compounds known as PCBs cannot be separated from the problem of solid waste, which we consider in chapter 5. PCBs are believed to produce cancer in experimental animals, and they have been linked to reproductive disorders, kidney damage, liver ailments, and eye irritations in humans. In 1968, some 10,000 people in Japan became ill after consuming rice oil contaminated with PCBs. Because of widespread contamination from manufacturing plants, especially those making transformers and capacitors, the manufacture of PCBs is now prohibited in the United States and the EPA has banned any discharge of PCBs into U.S. waters. The problem,

FIGURE 4.4
Oil Spills and Wildlife

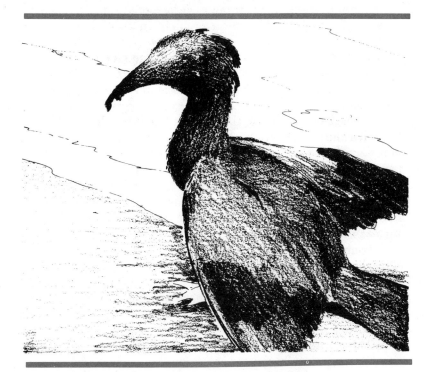

While oil spills have many harmful effects, birds are often among their most immediate and visible victims. Unable to maintain their body temperature once their plumage is covered with oil, many die of hypothermia. Survivors of the immediate spill may die subsequently as a result of eating contaminated fish and worms, or starve to death because their food supply has been destroyed.

Did You Know That . . .

According to the Congressional Research Service, approximately 10 percent of the nation's 1.4 million underground gasoline and oil storage tanks have leaks.

though, as in the case of other pollutants, is that it may take decades to clear up the contamination resulting from previous assaults on our water supply.

Pesticides and fertilizers are also important organic water pollutants. Much like PCBs, both were used extensively before any hazards were suspected. They ran off from farmlands into rivers and lakes, they were washed out of the air by rainfall, they were dumped into nearby bodies of water. Although it has long been banned in this country, **DDT** is found in many U.S. waters in extremely high concentrations. Droughts lower water levels and raise the concentration of the contaminants in the water that

DDT: The common abbreviation for the chemical name of a colorless, crystalline, organic pesticide (dichloro-diphenyl-trichloro-ethane), first used in 1939, that disorganizes the nervous systems of a variety of insects on contact; because of its toxic effects on other forms of wildlife, all nonessential uses of DDT have been banned in the United States and many other countries.

Nitrate(s): The name applied to any member of two groups of compounds derived from nitric acid, known as nitric acid esters and nitric acid salts; also refers to fertilizers containing potassium nitrate or sodium nitrate.

Typhoid fever: An infectious disease contracted by eating food or drinking water contaminated with the bacterium *Salmonella typhosa;* the first symptom is usually severe headache, which is followed by fever, diarrhea or constipation, loss of appetite, and may progress to delirium; typhoid fever usually clears up within 4 weeks but can be fatal if left untreated.

Asiatic cholera: An infection of the small intestine caused by the bacterium *Vibria cholerae* that results in severe, watery diarrhea, and in acute cases can lead to rapid dehydration and death if untreated; long confined to portions of South Asia, the disease has spread throughout the rest of the Third World and to the Gulf Coast of the United States since the 1950s.

Coliform bacteria: Any of several species of bacteria that inhabit the large intestine, and whose presence in water is an indicator of pollution from human waste.

remains. Unfortunately, many industries that dump treated wastes into waterways rely on dilution by ample water supplies to complete the purification process.

Nitrates are another organic water pollutant of increasing concern. These are primarily a problem in rural areas, where they contaminate the groundwater supply. The major sources of nitrate contamination are fertilizers, sewage sludge, and septic tanks. In addition, nitrates find their way into the water supply when ammonia released from manure is partly discharged into the atmosphere and partly converted by soil microbes into soluble nitrates in the soil, making them a significant problem in areas of intensive animal farming. [12] A recent EPA study estimated that more than half the nation's wells have water contaminated with nitrates, although only 2.4 percent were found to have levels that pose a health concern. [13] Nitrates appear to have the most serious effect on infants, whose stomachs apparently do not yet produce enough acid to prevent the growth of bacteria that convert nitrates to highly toxic nitrites.

Waterborne Diseases

Water supplies may also be contaminated by organisms that cause disease. This was one of the many discoveries made by Hippocrates, the ancient Greek physician who was the first to suspect that water could carry disease. He suggested that water be boiled or filtered before being consumed. Among diseases that may be transmitted by water contaminated by bacteria, viruses, or protozoa are typhoid and cholera, gastroenteritis, paratyphoid fever, and infectious hepatitis.

Typhoid fever and **Asiatic cholera**, diseases that attack and affect the human intestinal tract, are particularly dangerous. If typhoid- or cholera-infected waste finds its way into the water supply, the result can be an epidemic. In the famous 1854 case involving a pump on Broad Street in the London parish of St. James, 700 people died in a 17-week epidemic of cholera. Chicago discharged municipal wastes directly into Lake Michigan until well into the 20th century. Not surprisingly, typhoid fever was endemic in that area. [14]

Since it would be an impossible task to test water supplies for all possible disease-causing organisms, municipalities test for **coliform bacteria** as an indicator. These do not generally cause disease but are found naturally in the intestines of all warm-blooded animals, including humans. However, if they are present in concentrations of more than 4 per 100-milliliter sample, it suggests that the water supply may be contaminated by untreated

FIGURE 4.5
A Court for King Cholera

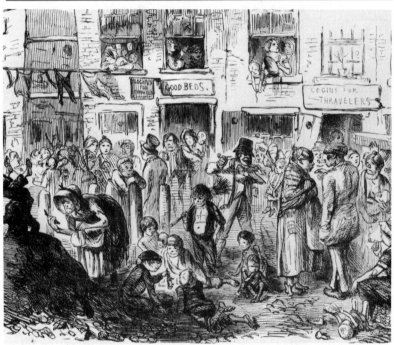

Source: Bettmann/Hulton.

This cartoon from the English periodical *Punch* depicts some of the living conditions that existed at the time of the great cholera epidemic of 1854. It is easy to see how the water supply could have been contaminated.

sewage and, therefore, unsafe for human consumption. Boating is permitted in water containing up to 10,000 coliforms per 100 milliliters but, as they say, don't fall in!

ENSURING SAFE DRINKING WATER

Half of the drinking water in the United States is obtained from rivers and other surface waterways; it can be contaminated by sewage, acid rain, pesticides, and nuclear or industrial waste. The other half comes from wells and underground reserves

Table 4.1 Coliform Bacteria and Water Use

Coliform Level	Activity Permitted
1 coliform or fewer per 100 milliliters of water	Water safe for drinking
4 coliforms or more per 100 milliliters of water	State must be notified and corrective action taken
2300 coliforms or fewer per 100 milliliters of water	Swimming is allowed
10,000 coliforms or fewer per 100 milliliters of water	Boating is allowed

Source: Environmental Protection Agency.

Federal Environmental Protection Agency standards for water use are based on coliform bacteria levels. These stipulate that municipal drinking water supplies must contain no more than 1 coliform per 100 milliliters of water. A coliform level of 4 or greater means that the supplier must notify state authorities and take corrective action.

(aquifers) that can be tainted by substances that leach from landfills, by toxic wastes, and by leaks from underground oil or other storage tanks. Researchers at Cornell University determined that over 60 percent of wells in rural areas contain unsafe levels of at least one substance. [15] The classic case of water pollution comes from Woburn, Massachusetts, an industrial suburb 12 miles from Boston. A mysterious series of deaths and illnesses over a period of 20 years finally led to a landmark court case in which victims of pollution sued those they felt were responsible. Indeed, well tests found various industrial solvents that are known to cause cancer in laboratory animals; the solvents were traced to a cleaning process at a W. R. Grace plant, and the wells were shut down—*after* doing their damage. Although the complicated trial ended in a settlement, the findings put both industries and homeowners on notice that each of us has a responsibility to monitor the quality of our water supply as well as maintain our own wellness. [16]

The first attempts at filtering water through sand beds to purify it for drinking occurred in 1872. Poughkeepsie, New York, became the first city in the United States to install sand filters to purify water. In the ensuing 20 years, the full potential of sand filters was recognized. [17] The Poughkeepsie filters were still in operation over 100 years later in 1977.

The origins of **chlorination** are even more recent. In 1908, the badly polluted condition of the local water supply prompted a court order to the private firm responsible for supplying water to Jersey City, New Jersey. Under court order to provide water that was safe for human consumption, the firm used calcium hypochlorite to destroy the harmful bacteria found in its water. The experiment was successful. Now sanctioned by law, the use of the chlorination process to purify water quickly spread throughout the United States. Today chlorination is used to purify most public water supplies in the United States.

Sand filters and chlorination are techniques used to ensure that public water supplies are safe for human consumption. The other side of the coin is ensuring that the water we use is as clean as possible when returned to the environment. This is the function of sewage-treatment plants, most of which are owned by local municipalities. (See Figure 4.6.) The first stage of sewage treatment is designed to remove the larger suspended solids through screening and sedimentation. This is usually followed by a secondary level of treatment in which bacteria and fungi are used to break down organic materials into their inorganic components (carbon dioxide, water, and minerals). In some instances, yet a third level of treatment is necessary. This may involve the use of techniques such as chemical coagulation or ion exchange. Since the average American generates approximately 100 gallons of wastewater daily, it is not surprising that sewage treatment is an increasingly large item in the budgets of many municipalities.

It is also an increasingly large problem. An estimated 75 percent of small municipalities in the United States do not meet federal water standards. Because the cost of conventional sewage-treatment plants is beyond the means of many of these communities, there have been a number of recent efforts to seek low-cost alternatives. In one such experiment, the Tennessee Valley Authority (TVA) has been assisting towns to create artificial wetlands. The TVA scheme is based on the fact that shallow marshes are natural purifying systems that can cleanse water of many harmful substances. In these planned lagoons, organisms in the water break down solid waste, plants absorb harmful substances created by the breakdown of nitrogen and phosphorous compounds, and clean water filters through a pond and the surrounding meadow grass and then into the stream or river that carries the naturally treated water downstream. [18]

Did You Know That . . .

Seven out of 10 Americans drink chlorinated water.

Chlorination: A widely used water purification process that involves the addition of a chlorine compound to disinfect drinking-water supplies.

FIGURE 4.6
Sewage Treatment Plant

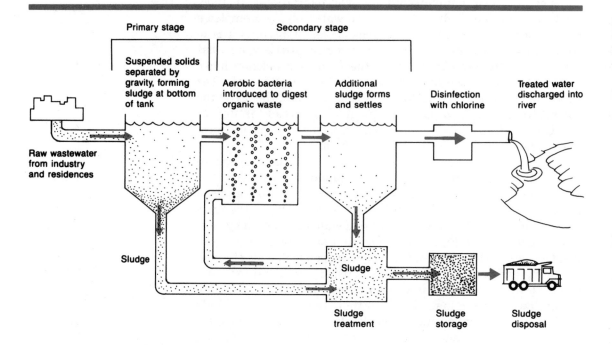

Source: Robert Italiano.

Wastewater generated by industry and residences contains a variety of contaminants. Sewage treatment plants such as the one depicted above remove or neutralize many of these contaminants via a multistage process. In the first or primary stage, most suspended solids are removed from the water by gravity in a settling tank. In the secondary stage, also called the biological treatment stage, bacteria are used to break down the remaining organic material. The water is then usually disinfected with chlorine before being discharged into a nearby river or other body of water. The treatment process generates sludge which is then disposed of in a variety of ways.

With widespread public concern about the safety of public water supplies, it is to be expected that shady entrepreneurs would step in to capitalize on these fears by offering to sell equipment that is usually expensive and may be unnecessary. *Consumer Reports,* for example, recently reported that although home water treatment is still in its infancy, it has attracted some 400 different manufacturers and their sales are expected to top $1 billion by 1995. [19]

(continued on p. 83)

Cleansing Waters

It is a tender spring morning in Benton, Kentucky (population 4,600). At the edge of a marsh, red-winged blackbirds call to each other from stands of cattails. A harlequin-faced wood duck dives beneath the shallow waters, turtles skid as they chase minnows, and the westerly breeze brings the scents of blackberry blossoms, wild iris and damp clay soil.

Welcome to Benton's sewage treatment facility. Every day, up to 1 million gallons of waste water are treated here—without machines, generators or engineers. The lagoon and three adjacent marshes naturally break down pollution. They return to the Clarks River a stream that is clean beyond waste water treatment standards set by the Environmental Protection Agency. Benton's wetlands are a model for small towns that need clean water, cheaply.

In 1985 Benton was facing bankruptcy. For years the town had violated the Clean Water Act, relying on an antiquated waste water treatment facility built for 330,000 gallons a day but besieged with more than 500,000. The water that ran into Clarks River surpassed federal limits for suspended solids, ammonia, nitrogen and bacteria. That year the EPA notified Benton that its permit under the Clean Water Act was about to be revoked, so the town would face $10,000 in daily fines. A new plant would cost as much as $3 million.

It's a common dilemma. Nearly three-quarters of all communities under 10,000 violate federal water quality standards. Small cities not only have fewer funds but often discharge waste into smaller streams that get polluted more quickly. Ironically, those same towns often depend on water-based tourism like boating and fishing.

'Enter the Tennessee Valley Authority (TVA), with a proposal to study the effectiveness of using "artificial" wetlands as a means of sewage treatment. The TVA had already planted wetland systems at coal mines to treat acid drainage, with huge success; now it was assisting towns with wetland design for sewer systems. With partial funding from the TVA, Benton hired a local engineer, who for $260,000 built an EPA-approved wetlands system to treat 1 million gallons of waste water a day. "What we paid for our wetland would have covered only the cost of the engineering fee on a conventional mechanical plant," says Gayle Frye, Benton's grants coordinator.

Wetlands work because shallow marshes are powerful, natural water-cleansing systems, full of microbial organisms, insects and aquatic animals that decompose wastes and recycle water. A typical design consists of four stages: a settling pond, marsh, pond and meadow.

■ Untreated waste water empties into a settling pond where oxygen supports organisms that break down solid waste.

■ A marsh then supplies a natural filter of cattails and bulrush, where microbes feed off nitrogen and phosphorus, breaking them down to substances readily absorbed by plants.

■ Water, now fed with the oxygen that adheres in a thin film to the plant roots, moves to the third stage, a pond. Algae feed on any remaining nutrients as the clean water flows through a filter of meadow grasses into a stream. Stream water, cleaner than most municipally treated water, supports fish, aquatic wildlife and birds.

Wetland designs differ from town to town, depending on size, soil and climate; a dozen or so systems are now being built across the country. They do require some land, about one acre for every 50,000 gallons of daily waste water; a town of 10,000 people, for example, needs to set aside about 20 wetland acres. Once a wetland is established, it practically takes care of itself. In Benton, one person, Daniel Lane, monitors water levels and quality, and mows the lawn. Whatever the wetland design, no matter where it is, one thing is clear: the water that comes out of it.

Source: M. Klockenbrink, *American Health* (September 1989), p. 72.

Home Water Purifiers: How to Make a Rational Purchase

"Congratulations!!! You are absolutely guaranteed to receive one of our top five fabulous prizes."

So promised the postcard that Terry Hudson of Calabasaf, California, got last July. When he called the long-distance number printed on the postcard, a voice on the other end screamed in apparent excitement, "My God!!! You've got one of the top numbers! It's the 1990 Chrysler convertible!"

There was just one little string attached. When Terry called back to claim his car, the phone rep launched into a pitch for a *water filter.* "They told me the filter would remove minerals and all kinds of contaminants, down to the microgram." Terry was informed he'd have to purchase a filter to guarantee his prize. The charge: $493, for a unit whose retail value is actually $50 to $75, according to Federal Trade Commission attorneys. Terry Hudson did receive the filter, but never the prize.

Nationwide, reports of deceitful tactics used to sell water filters are increasing. Telemarketing with promised but never-delivered prizes is one tactic. Another is to convince customers that their water is unsafe to drink. To raise a false alarm about water pollution, peddlers from a California water-filter company went door-to-door clad in doctor's smocks and armed with clippings about toxic-waste dumps. Solicitors from a Maryland company collected water samples from homeowners and returned later with phony lab results that they claimed proved the water was unsafe.

Erik Olson, an attorney who monitors drinking-water regulations for the National Wildlife Federation, says that the NWF has "a real concern with the scare tactics being used" to sell these treatment units. He and other experts I surveyed—including professors, EPA officials, and water-utility spokesmen—warn that some devices sold as cure-alls for polluted water are useless.

There *are* legitimate water-treatment devices on the market. . . . To find one, though, you have to navigate your way through a sea of deliberate overstatement and confusion. The first step is simply to find out exactly what *is* in your tap water.

How Safe Is Tap Water?

In theory, the 85% of us who draw our water from public supplies (the other 15% own private wells) should feel our water is safe, because federal law regulates public water supplies. The Safe Drinking Water Act requires that water utilities provide treatment to guard against 83 priority contaminants. In practice, however, the Safe Drinking Water Act may be no guarantee of safety. One big problem is that the Environmental Protection Agency, charged with enforcing the Act, rarely prosecutes violators. According to NWF Attorney Olson, the EPA took no civil actions against Safe Drinking Water Act offenders in all of 1989.

In part because of the EPA's lax enforcement, contaminants occasionally slip through municipal utilities' treatment processes. In one notorious drinking-water pollution case, 19 children in Woburn, Massachusetts, died of leukemia. Scientists linked the deaths to two industrial solvents, trichloroethylene and perchloroethylene, which had leaked into community wells.

Just how widespread illness caused by drinking-water contamination is, nobody knows. Experts tend to play down the prevalence of cancer-causing industrial chemicals in water. Says Al Stevens, a director of the EPA's Office of Drinking Water, "The risk of getting cancer from drinking water is small. In fact, there's a controversy over whether it exists at all."

But episodes like Woburn do create legitimate cause for concern.

Testing Your Water

To find out whether your water is safe—and whether you need a filter—have your water tested by an independent lab. Call your state health department for recommendations. . . .

Heed this caution: *Do not* invite a filter salesperson to your house to do a "free" water test, as advertised in the phone book. The test that salespeople typically offer is like a hocus-pocus magic show: It's meant to mystify you, but it won't tell you whether life-threatening contaminants have infiltrated your water.

One favorite "free test" goes like this: Salesperson fills a test tube with your water, then adds a chemical. Presto! Your water turns yellow. Or maybe sediment forms. Salesperson says, "Serious contamination! Your water turned yellow." Or, acting dismayed, "Look at all those unhealthy solids!" What they don't tell you is that the change in the water sample was caused by the chemical reacting with chlorine (used nationwide to disinfect water) or with harmless minerals (which precipitate as sediment). According to such "tests," there's not a tap in the country that delivers safe water.

The Likely Suspects

Hundreds of toxins have been identified in drinking water over the years. How do you know which contaminants to test for? Here are the most likely suspects:

• **LEAD:** Lead can leach into your water from lead service pipes or lead/tin solder in copper plumbing (illegal as of 1986). In the low levels found in water, lead can cause learning disabilities in children. Lead may be *the* most common drinking-water contaminant, affecting one in six households. Buy a treatment unit if tests reveal a lead concentration above 10 micrograms/L.

• **TRIHALOMETHANES:** Trihalomethanes (THMs) form when chlorine, used for disinfection, reacts with decayed vegetation naturally present in the water. One familiar THM is chloroform; it and other THMs cause cancer in lab animals. If your utility draws its water from a river, lake, or reservoir, you will be exposed to THMs, especially during fall, when decayed vegetation abounds. What level of THMs is "safe" is a matter that the EPA is debating; current regulations require a total THM concentration less than 100 micrograms/L.

• **NITRATE:** Contamination with nitrate, a product of chemical fertilizers, is the most common reason for closing wells in agricultural areas. Its primary danger is to infants: It causes an illness called "blue-baby syndrome," which leads to suffocation. If you are hooked up to a large water utility, you're probably safe from nitrate, since most utilities are conscientious about nitrate testing. The EPA's "safe" limit on nitrate is 10 mg/L.

• **RADON:** Unlike many contaminants, radon is present in water through no fault of human endeavor; it's a naturally occurring radioactive gas formed from uranium. You are most at risk of radon exposure if your water source is a private well or small utility (serving fewer than 500 people) in Maine, New Hampshire, Connecticut, North Carolina, or Arizona. If your water comes from a surface source (river, lake, or reservoir), don't worry! The radon will escape into the air before the water reaches your tap. Radon is hazardous at concentrations above 10,000 picocuries/L.

• **VOLATILE ORGANIC COMPOUNDS:** The term volatile organic compounds (VOCs) encompasses an array of chemicals used for varied purposes: as degreasers in industry, for dry cleaning, for household spot remover, for air freshener, even in food processing. VOCs migrate easily from dump sites, through the soil, into the groundwater. (Two VOCs caused the leukemia deaths in Woburn.) Although experts say that VOCs are not as prevalent in water supplies as lead, nitrate, THMs, and radon, episodes like Woburn show that the consequences of VOC contamination are serious. You're at risk of VOC exposure only if you drink groundwater; VOCs evaporate quickly from surface water. If a VOC shows up in your water, call the EPA's drinking-water hotline [800-426-4791] to find out if the level is dangerous.

• **PESTICIDES:** If you live in an agricultural area, you're at risk of pesticide exposure. In Suffolk County, New York, for instance, a state survey documented that 2,000 private wells were contaminated with aldicarb. As with VOCs, call the EPA's drinking water hotline if tests uncover pesticides in your water.

That's what *might* be in your water, besides two Hs and an O.

Before you rush to the post office to mail your water samples, you can save money by requesting a copy of your municipal utility's water analysis. For example, the Montgomery County,

Maryland, utility publishes a free list of the contaminants they test for, along with the yearly average concentration of each, the maximum monthly average, and the EPA limit. Montgomery County's list shows that there are no pesticides in the water, so folks there needn't bother testing for pesticides.

There are two contaminants your utility cannot tell you about: lead and THMs. That's because lead leaches into your water on its way from the water treatment plant to your home. So, although the lead level may be zero at your water utility, the level at your tap could be hazardous. Likewise, THMs form en route to your tap, as chlorine combines slowly with invisible molecules from decayed vegetation.

The Units That Cure

With luck (and probability) on your side, tests will show that your water is safe. If not, the cure is a system that's designed specifically to remove the contaminants that surfaced in the tests.

• CAUTION: Research this purchase carefully, like you would the purchase of a car. Water-treatment devices aren't subject to EPA regulation, so quality control is a serious problem. Some shoddily manufactured units have little effect against pollutants. Others can *add* contaminants to your water. For example, glue in Norelco's "Clean Water Machine" leaked methylene chloride into water flowing through the system. Norelco, fully aware of the hazard, marketed the machine for five years, until a federal judge barred its further sale in 1988. Environmental engineers have documented similar problems with other filters: Some contain plastics that taint the water with VOCs; others contain residues of hazardous solvents.

When shopping for a water-treatment system, your best guarantee against slipshod manufacturing is to buy a system that's been tested by an independent lab. One lab that certifies filter performance is the National Sanitation Foundation (NSF) [313-769-8010]. Consumers Union has also run tests.

Here are the four most common water-treatment systems, with descriptions of what contaminants

each removes and the experts' recommendations for lab-tested brands:

• CARBON FILTERS: Carbon filters are best for extracting THMs, VOCs, radon, and pesticides. They're powerless against lead, other metals, and nitrate. The active ingredient is "activated carbon," a charcoal-like substance with millions of pores to soak up chemicals. The more carbon the filter contains, the better. Faucet-mount filters are ineffective because they contain so little carbon: select a larger unit that mounts under the sink or sits on the counter.

When the carbon fills up with contaminants, you'll need to change the filter cartridge. There's no way to see when the carbon is full. A safe rule of thumb is to change the cartridge every couple of months, according to Dr. Vern Snoeyink, a University of Illinois professor who studies these systems. *Don't* believe manufacturers' claims that the carbon can last years, says Dr. Snoeyink.

A system whose performance both the NSF and Consumers Union have verified is the Amway E-9230, which retails for $200.

• REVERSE-OSMOSIS UNITS: Reverse-osmosis units are the best solution to lead and nitrate contamination. They remove *some* THMs, VOCs, and pesticides, but are useless against radon.

These devices contain coiled plastic sheets, called "semi-permeable membranes," which strain out contaminants. One drawback is that they waste water. Only 10 to 25 percent of the influent water passes through the strainer; the rest goes down the drain along with the contaminants.

One unit tested by both the NSF and Consumers Union is the Culligan Aqua-Cleer H-83, which hides under your sink; various versions retail for $600 to $1,000. Another is the counter-top Shaklee BestWater System 50800, for $275.

• DISTILLERS: Distillers remove lead and other metals. They operate by boiling the water, then condensing the steam and dripping it into a jug. Anything that doesn't evaporate with the boiling water stays behind. Don't buy a distiller if your problem is VOCs, THMs, or radon; these volatilize along with the steam.

The major quality-control problem with distillers is that some corrode. Two that resist corrosion are the Aqua Clean Model 4 ($299) and the

Sears 34555 ($150), both tested by Consumers Union.

• ION-EXCHANGE SOFTENERS: Water softeners, developed 60 years ago, are the oldest home water-treatment technology. Their primary function is not to eliminate health-threatening chemicals, but to remove harmless calcium and magnesium, which prevent soap from lathering and create scale in your teapot. Softeners can also intercept radioactive radium and barium, but *don't* let a salesman talk you into buying one to remove lead, VOCs, radon, or any of the other contaminants mentioned above.

According to Consumers Union, almost all softeners do the job they were designed for; choose one based on convenience and design. The average cost is $1,000.

Final Words of Advice

For combinations of contaminants, your only solution may be to install both a carbon filter and a reverse-osmosis unit. For instance, if your water contains lead and THMs, you'll want reverse osmosis to take out the lead, and carbon to guarantee that no THMs escape. Also, both reverse-osmosis units and carbon filters work best if you install a sediment filter ahead of them to prevent clogging. Buy one at a plumbing store for about $40.

Remember: Don't believe your water is unsafe just because someone wearing a white coat knocks at your door and tells you so. Don't panic if your water coagulates when a saleswoman drops a chemical into it. And, please, don't buy your water filter from a telemarketer.

Federal Trade Commission attorney Jane Alcock, who's suing the telemarketer that defrauded Terry Hudson, says, "You wouldn't believe how many *really intelligent* people fall for this sort of thing." You wouldn't believe it—until it happens to you.

Source: J. MacDonald, *Garbage* (March/April 1991), pp. 31–35.

Home water-treatment systems come in several varieties. Carbon-treatment systems use charcoal filters to trap contaminants. These units may attach to a faucet or may be connected to the supply for the whole house. Distillation systems heat tap water to the boiling level and then cool the resulting steam. The "purified" water (condensed steam) is then routed on and the contaminants remain behind. There is also a reverse-osmosis unit, in which water is forced through a kind of film that traps most chemical molecules.

Before purchasing such a system, it is best to proceed with caution. Such systems are usually not needed where municipally treated water is available and may themselves cause as many problems as they protect against, especially if not maintained properly. At a minimum, you should take the time to find out whether the unit you are considering meets National Sanitation Foundation standards. And you should be on the alert for shady door-to-door selling tactics that are increasingly common to the home water-treatment industry. For further information, see "Home Water Purifiers," above.

(continued on p. 85)

Making a Difference: What One Person Can Do

1. First things first: Never flush toxics of any kind down sinks or toilets. This includes disinfectants, most household cleansers, and solvents of any type. Keep in mind that anything you do flush away may come back out of your tap.

2. Have your tap water tested for lead and other contaminants. Most local utilities will do it for a small fee, or you can hire a private tester. Tested or untested, if a faucet hasn't been used for six hours or longer, let cold water run through the pipes for five seconds to two minutes to clear any potentially dangerous sediment sitting in the pipes.

3. Use only water from the cold water tap for drinking, cooking, and making baby formula. Hot water is likely to contain higher levels of lead.

4. Flush and clear sediment from your water heater every six months or so. If you go on vacation and it's not been used, run the hot water when you come back to flush any build-up.

5. For more information on drinking water contaminants, call the EPA's toll-free safe drinking-water hotline, 800-426-4791, to help with interpretations of the law and its enforcement.

6. The Safe Drinking Water Act requires monitoring of community water systems that have 14 or more service connections. If you have questions about your water, records of such monitoring should be available from your local environmental or health departments. For information about the quality of local water call your local village/city manager, or the state agency in charge of regulating public water supplies. If you are in a community water system, ask your supplier if the system contains lead piping. If the answer is yes, ask if it's being replaced. Drinking water can be treated at the plant to make it less corrosive for an annual cost of less than one dollar per person.

7. [To limit] freshwater pollution: Conserve, conserve, conserve. The less water used, the less demand worldwide, the less risk of contamination. Also make sure toilets and showerheads are the most efficient available.

8. The sale of bottled water continues to grow 15 to 20 percent a year. Worldwide, we consume 5.7 gallons of bottled water per person each year. For a rating of the dozens available, check out *Consumer Reports,* January 1987.

9. Water-purification systems for your tap are another option. But be careful. There are dozens on the market, each with a specific cleansing purpose. And there are as many hoodwinking purification systems salesmen as there are systems. They'll promise anything and deliver little. Careful investigation is an absolute. Try *Consumer Reports* for recommendations.

10. Buy organically grown fruits and vegetables. As the demand for organic foods grows, pesticide use will eventually lessen—the better for both groundwater and consumers.

11. The U.S. Public Interest Research Group (USPIRG) publishes "Testing for Toxics: A Guide to Investigating Drinking Water Quality," which discusses relatively easy methods for communities or individuals to use to test their water for contamination. Write USPIRG, 215 Pennsylvania Ave. SE, Washington, DC 20003, for a copy.

12. The Izaak Walton League of America operates an extensive national volunteer program called "Save Our Streams." The league encourages community groups to adopt an area of a stream, remove debris, replant vegetation, and monitor water quality.

13. Use unbleached (non-white) and undyed paper products whenever possible, for two reasons. First, the dioxins involved in the manufacture of bleached papers are primary polluters of rivers; second, dyed toilet paper and paper towels carry more pollutants into the water.

14. Ask at your car wash if they recycle their water. If they don't, find another washer. If you wash your car at home; be sure and turn the hose off when you're not rinsing.

15. Many brands of toothpaste contain cadmium (which becomes harmful as large quantities of it are released into the groundwater) but manufacturers are not required by the FDA to list

it among the active ingredients. Write to the maker of your brand and ask whether it uses cadmium. If it does, pick a new brand.

16. Use "gray water" (i.e., water previously used, like dishwater or a pet's drinking water) or rain water for plants and garden, or use an underground drip irrigation system in the garden to send water directly to the roots without evaporation or wastage.

17. If you have a small garden, use water-soluble fertilizers. Available at most hardware and garden stores, they are absorbed almost immediately by roots and leaves. They don't dissolve in the soil and then leach into groundwater.

18. Ask at your local nursery about which plants will grow in your area with little or no watering.

19. Don't hose down your sidewalk or driveway, sweep it.

20. If you live near contaminated water, contact Clean Water Action (317 Pennsylvania Ave. SE, Washington, DC 20003, 202-547-1196). The group uses such reports to twist the arms of congresspeople into action. They are also a good source for information about how to get involved.

21. Under the Clean Water Act, anyone who discharges pollutants into a waterway must have a permit that spells out exactly what they are allowed to discharge. Every month, the company must report to the EPA or to the state on its compliance or non-compliance with the terms of that permit. The law also allows for citizens to take direct action against those companies. Several lawsuits have been originated, fought, and won against major companies based on citizen complaints. If you have a complaint, contact an office of the Natural Resources Defense Council, the local EPA, or another environmental group.

Source: W. Steger and J. Bowermaster, *Saving the Earth: A Citizen's Guide to Environmental Action* (New York: A. A. Knopf, 1990), pp. 211–212.

It seems fitting to close our discussion of water with a comment from the world's foremost authority on water, Jacques Cousteau.

No part of an ocean [or any body of water] can be fenced off for the use and abuse of a single country, and the actions of any nation inevitably affect the ocean all of us need and use.... The ocean conceals the most formidable potential resources of our planet. But to tackle them—to accept this challenge—we must think big, think unselfishly, think globally, and think far ahead. [20] 𝖂

5

The Waste Stream

New Yorkers are building an architectural wonder on Staten Island. When completed in the late 1990s, this conical-shaped structure will be taller and heavier than the largest of Egypt's pyramids. The ancient Egyptians built their pyramids out of huge stone blocks. On Staten Island, the construction material is the garbage of 9 million New Yorkers. [1]

PERHAPS YOU SQUEEZE the last bit of shampoo out of the container as you listen to the news on the battery-powered waterproof radio. You unwrap clothing fresh from the dry-cleaner. You reach over the morning newspaper for a bottle of juice and then a jug of milk for the cereal you pour from a box. As you wipe up a spill with a paper towel, you are, within the first half-hour of the day, well on your way to producing the nearly 4 pounds of garbage that is on average generated by each American daily.

MASSES OF DISCARDS

What we throw away literally mounts up. Residents of New York City discard 24,000 tons of material each day. At 3.5 pounds per person per day, New Yorkers throw out roughly 9 times their own body weight in rubbish each year, 2 times as much per person as

FIGURE 5.1
The Throwaway Society

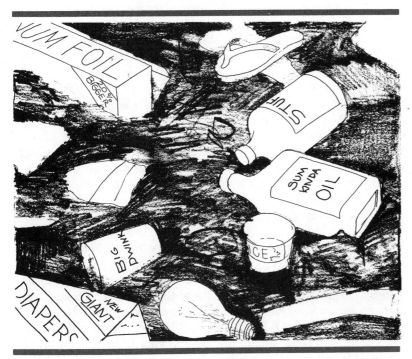

According to the Environmental Protection Agency, the volume of municipal solid waste generated each day in this country increased from 2.7 pounds per person in 1960 to 4 pounds per person by 1988. Current EPA projections are that by the year 2000 this figure will rise to 4.4 pounds per person per day for a daily total of 216 million tons.

Did You Know That . . .

One of the largest waste dumps in the world is Fresh Kills landfill on Staten Island in New York. Fresh Kills receives 17,000 tons of refuse from New York City each day, six days a week. It covers 3,000 acres and takes up 2.4 billion cubic feet of space.

residents of Hamburg or Rome and up to 4 times more per person than those who live in Manila. While New Yorkers are notorious for their ability to generate trash, the national picture is only slightly better. Americans generate an estimated 160 to 200 million tons of solid waste annually, at least 80 percent more than in 1960. [2]

But solid waste is only part of the waste-disposal problem. Equally important, perhaps more so in terms of its potential health effects, is the problem of toxic waste. American industry currently produces 250 million tons of toxic wastes annually. Less than 50 percent of such chemicals are being disposed of safely, according to the EPA. The rest is illegally dumped in municipal landfills, open pits, or lagoons. The disposal options dwindle daily as landfills fill and citizens contest even legal dumping. Meanwhile, water and air continue to be polluted. There *is* encouraging news, however, because this is an environmental concern that individuals *can* tackle. But it should be noted that it took some fairly dramatic events to turn the tide of the waste stream.

There was, for example, the voyage of the freighter *Pelicano*. Like the *Flying Dutchman,* the *Pelicano* seemed condemned to sail the seas endlessly as it tried for 2 years to unload 14,000 tons of toxic incinerator ash it had taken on in Philadelphia in September 1986. After repeatedly failing to find a port where its cargo would be accepted, the *Pelicano* illegally dumped 4,000 pounds off a Haitian beach in October 1988. A month later, the *Pelicano*'s voyage ended in Singapore, where the captain announced that he had unloaded the ash in a country he refused to name. [3]

Two years earlier, there was the saga of the New York town of Islip's wandering garbage scow *Mobro*. Loaded with more than 3,000 tons of Long Island refuse, it was turned away by ports as far away as Belize before returning to New York. There its cargo was finally incinerated, and the resulting 400 tons of ash wound up in the landfill that had been the first of many to reject the *Mobro*'s cargo. [4] The moral of these tales? What is tossed out must go *somewhere*! Each year, Americans throw away 16 billion disposable diapers, 1.6 billion pens, 2 billion razors and blades, and 220 million tires. We discard enough aluminum to rebuild the entire U.S. commercial airline fleet every 3 months. [5] Not including sludge and construction wastes, American household waste annually is enough to spread 30 stories high over 1,000 football fields—enough to fill a bumper-to-bumper convoy of garbage trucks halfway to the moon. And we are running out of dumping space worldwide. In the United States, more than 50 percent of the existing landfills will be closed within a few years, and the attempts to create new landfills or to expand old ones are met with the NIMBY reflex (Not In My Back Yard). NIMBY has been joined by GOOMBY (Get Out Of My Back Yard) and LULU (Locally Undesirable Land Use). As the battle wages on, each side needs to examine facts, actions, and consequences.

SOLID WASTE: WHERE DOES IT ALL COME FROM?

Garbage anthropologists say that the average American household is an around-the-clock, multiproduct trash factory generat-

FIGURE 5.2
What We Throw Away: A Breakdown by Weight

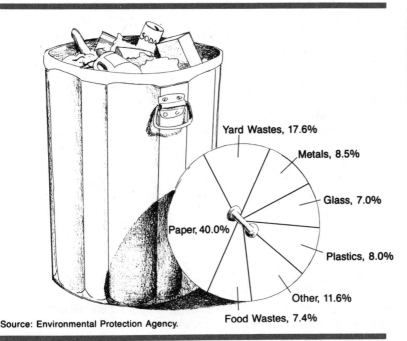

Source: Environmental Protection Agency.

Did You Know That . . .

A total of 15 million tons of solid waste was shipped from one state to another in the United States in 1989. New Jersey accounted for 53 percent of the total amount shipped (7.5 million tons) and New York for 16 percent (2.4 million tons).

According to 1988 figures from the Environmental Protection Agency, the single largest component of the municipal solid waste stream is paper and paper products, which account for 40 percent of all solid waste by weight. The remaining 60 percent consists of yard wastes, metals, plastic, food wastes, glass, and other.

ing 87.5 gallons each week. [6] We throw away 3 times as much as our grandparents did when they were our age, largely because they simply did not have the volume of plastic bottles, cans, old appliances, broken toys, newspapers, magazines, and the ever-present junk mail, automobile equipment, labor-saving devices and solutions, or even the same amount of food scraps and lawn clippings.

In the United States today, packaging materials of all types are estimated to be between 30 and 40 percent, by weight, of the municipal refuse and make up perhaps half of the volume of household waste. An empty plastic grocery bag weighs almost nothing, but somehow we manage to throw away an amount equal to 216 million pounds of them each year; $1 in every $10 spent on food goes to pay for its packaging. There is more to all this than throwing money away. The useful life of most of what we throw away is also a far cry from grandma and grandpa's young days. A steel or aluminum can is used only once before it may be dropped into the garbage. Throwing away that container after a single use is an extremely wasteful practice. This wastes as much energy as pouring out a half gallon of gasoline. [7]

Not all solid wastes originate with households or industries. Agricultural activities, for example, produce more than 1.8 billion tons of waste each year. About three quarters of this is manure, which is piled in dumps, from where it pollutes streams and waterways. In addition, mining operations produce about 1.35 billion tons of debris a year. Most of this material is rock, dirt, sand, and slag that remains when metals are extracted from the earth. These piles, while ugly, may not represent a loss of valuable raw materials. They are, however, subject to erosion and a continuing source of acid pollutants that too often contaminate surfacewater and groundwater supplies. [8]

WHERE DOES IT GO?

When it comes to solid waste, what goes around comes around. A total of 160 million tons of solid waste has to go somewhere. And so it does—out of sight but not necessarily out of mind—as the troubled voyages of the *Pelicano* and the *Mobro* remind us. Where does it all go?

The options are limited. Once upon a time, not terribly long ago, in fact, the most popular option was the **open dump**. As recently as the 1950s and 1960s, many and perhaps most American towns featured a "town dump," which was the designated final resting place of solid waste from the local community. Here, usually on the outskirts of town, was deposited all unwanted solid waste. Garbage, paper products, used refrigerators, old bedsprings, and automobile tires, all found their way to the dump. Left exposed to the elements and the vagaries of time, they slowly (very slowly) faded away. For the most part, so too have open dumps, a victim of changing times, increasing concern about the environment, and a scarcity of open land.

The marine equivalent of the open dump is **ocean dumping**. Primarily an East Coast phenomenon and most often associated with New York, ocean dumping involves the use of barges to haul refuse to a designated location, usually a natural trench or canyon on the ocean floor. In this way, most of the trash is

Open dump: A place where solid waste (refuse, garbage, trash, and the like) is taken and left uncovered; also known as a dump site.

Ocean dumping: The practice of hauling solid waste into the ocean and dumping it in one or more locations.

(continued on p. 94)

Truckin' Trash

Ed Martin leans against his Peterbilt cabover, eyeing the 3,000-pound blocks of compacted garbage being fork-lifted onto its 42-foot-long tractor trailer. He had spent the previous night in his cab's sleeper berth at a Queens, N.Y., warehouse after hauling a load of steel bars from Ohio to New York City. Now, twenty minutes after backing into the loading area at the Star Recycling transfer station in Brooklyn, N.Y., Ed will point his giant rig westward for a 440-mile trip to the Willow Creek landfill outside of Atwater, Ohio (pop. 800).

On the road, only state transportation inspectors will know that his cargo is a 47,000-pound mass of used paper cups and soiled mattresses, shards of sheetrock, rotting banana peels, and other debris that's been picked clean of recyclables. At the Willow Creek dump, he'll join more than 90 other trucks that disgorge up to 1,900 tons of out-of-state garbage each day. A look of scorn creases Ed's weathered face as he anticipates the inspections at Pennsylvania weight stations ("they hassle you when they see it's garbage"), and the goatlike scent exuding from the rubbish after the 9-hour trek. "Garbage is the best paying freight around, but if I had my way, I'd be going back empty," he grouses.

Ed's massive rig is just one of the thousands of trucks long-hauling rubbish from the East Coast to the American heartland. Faced with soaring dumping fees and shrinking landfill space, in 1989 private carters in New York and New Jersey trucked 13.4 million tons of garbage over hundreds of miles into states like Indiana, Ohio, Pennsylvania, and Kentucky.

Every hour of every day in the year, about 43 tractor trailers, each burdened with about 20 tons of New Jersey's garbage, roll onto the state's roadways, bound for landfills scattered throughout the Midwest and the South. The cost to New Jersey taxpayers is enormous—Allen Moore, president of the National Solid Wastes Management Association (NSWMA), puts the figure at $700 million over the past six years.

Realizing that the East Coast's waste threatens to overwhelm the Midwest's landfill capacity, many states are legislating roadblocks to slow the influx of garbage. But midwestern and southern states are sending millions of tons of their own trash out on the road! Missouri estimates it ships 34 percent of its municipal solid waste to landfills in Kansas and Illinois. (Illinois also ships to Indiana, Kentucky, Michigan, and Wisconsin.)

All but 12 states are garbage importers *and* exporters. One reason for the waste trading is found in that oft-heard, overly simplistic lament: "We're running out of landfill space." Sure, some urban areas lack the land for burying or burning much of their waste, which is why, say, St. Louis and Kansas City, Mo., are scouting landfills in other states. But in a nation as vast as the U.S., there's plenty of open countryside for garbage disposal, which is why St. Louis and Kansas City can ship to facilities in Illinois and Kansas—even as four other states ship to Missouri.

"People here have got to realize that this is more than just a Midwest versus an East Coast issue," says Scott Holste of the Missouri Department of Natural Resources.

Guppies and Garbage, Protected Equally

To some degree, trucking garbage is a regional issue requiring regional cooperation. But to a great extent it really does pit the East Coast—specifically New York and New Jersey—against the rest of the country. Together, the two states were responsible for 53 percent of the estimated 15 million tons of waste shipped via the interstate system in 1989.

Southern and midwestern states seeking to stymie the invasion of imported garbage cannot turn to the federal government. The feds have virtually no control over the interstate movement of municipal solid waste. As the journal *Environmental Law* notes, " . . . every article of commercial activity (minnows, cantaloupes, scrap, timber, and yes, even garbage) is considered an article of commerce, and its interstate movement is constitutionally protected. . . ."

Ironically, a thwarted attempt by New Jersey to ban out-of-state trash from rolling into its *own* landfills has impeded other states from blockading New Jersey's waste. In the early 1970s, Philadelphia trucked most of its garbage to New Jersey's southern landfills. This appalled members of the New Jersey State Legislature, who passed a statute prohibiting waste importation. In 1978, the U.S. Supreme Court struck down the statute in a prophetic ruling: "Tomorrow, cities in New Jersey may find it necessary to send their waste into Pennsylvania or New York for disposal, and those states might claim the right to close their borders. The Commerce Clause will protect New Jersey in the future, just as it protects her neighbors now, from efforts by one state to isolate itself . . . from a problem shared by all."

Having closed more than 300 landfills over the past 20 years, which were either too polluted or just too full, New Jersey exported 5.5 million tons of garbage in 1989. And with only 11 regional landfills remaining and an ambitious, statewide recycling program that's still in its infancy, New Jersey's garbage exodus shows no sign of abating.

Farmers and miners scattered across rural counties turn up their noses at the garbage convoys that come rolling over their verdant hills. "People there think East Coast garbage is dirtier—filled with syringes and hazardous waste—and there's too much of it," says Scott Holste of Missouri's Department of Natural Resources.

[In 1990], seeking to waive the Commerce Clause, U.S. Sen. Dan Coats (R-Ind.) introduced legislation that would have enabled states to seal their borders to imported trash. The bill passed in the Senate by a 67 to 18 vote, but it was later "killed in conference by New Jersey's senators," says Tim Goeglein, a spokesman for Mr. Coats. "Indiana is tired of being the trash bin for New Jersey."

Ironically, had Mr. Coats' bill become law, it could have been used to stem the flow of *Indiana's* trash into Illinois, Kentucky, Michigan, and Ohio. And garbage bans would devastate towns in northern New Jersey and New York's Long Island, where the highway is the only way out for their growing mounds of rubbish.

New York City, however, has another disposal option—the gargantuan Fresh Kills landfill on Staten Island. Fresh Kills has a lifetime that extends into the next century. So why are the City's private carters sending more than 7 million tons of commercial garbage over hundreds of miles to distant landfills? Solely because in 1988, the City more than doubled its dumping fee at Fresh Kills to approximately $40 a cubic yard (roughly $120 a ton) for garbage collected from restaurants, construction companies, department stores, and other businesses.

"The City said it was trying to conserve space at Fresh Kills, when it was really trying to raise revenues," says Allen Moore of the NSWMA. "Overnight, the garbage-shipping industry was born."

Enticed by southern and midwestern dumping fees that average about $25 a ton, New York garbage brokers are converting empty warehouses and back lots into makeshift transfer stations where workers unload 25-yd. packer trucks (which pick up the City's commercial refuse), and load the waste onto tractor trailers for the long haul. "It's cheaper for me to send the garbage 1,000 miles away than it is to send it just a few miles to Fresh Kills," says Joe Bergeron, general manager of the Star Recycling transfer station in Brooklyn.

New York's two state inspectors are scrambling to keep track of the City's 183 (known) transfer stations. Glenn Milstrey of New York's Department of Environmental Conservation reports that inspectors are finding "numerous" environmental violations at many of the stations. Mr. Milstrey lists the Star Recycling transfer station as "one of the few that are [licensed]—they're one of the good guys."

Star Recycling is an $11 million operation covering five acres, hard by the Brooklyn waterfront.

Here, workers lean over conveyor belts that channel a constant stream of waste, pulling aluminum, metals, glass, cardboard, and high-grade paper from the 1,700 tons of garbage that roll into the facility each day. The rest of the garbage is sent packing, baled like hay. Each day, Star sends up to 80 tractor trailers, each laden with up to 23 tons of garbage, to landfills in Ohio, Indiana, West Virginia, and Georgia.

Every weekday, Star also railroads three boxcars laden with 270 tons of baled garbage to Lineville, Iowa, where workers unload the trash onto trucks bound for a privately owned landfill 55 miles across the Missouri border. Missouri officials call the landfill, near Trenton, a "sloppy operation." They're suing the landfill's owner, principally for failing to prevent contaminated rainwater from leaching through the dump and into a nearby creek.

Mr. Bergeron argues he wouldn't send waste to a dirty dump because, as the "garbage generator," Star Recycling might be held responsible for cleanup costs. Besides, until the lawsuit is settled, the Missouri landfill can legally continue accepting up to 3,000 tons of trash each week, regardless of where it comes from. And that angers Kathleen McCartney, a retired schoolteacher who lives nearby.

"We raise livestock here, and that landfill is leaking into our shallow well water," she says. "So what are we going to do—feed our cattle on bottled water?"

Responding to what she claims is an "inundation" of out-of-state garbage merchants seeking to build landfills in northern Missouri, Ms. McCartney has founded the Waste Information Network to help others in Missouri block imported garbage. "We're not opposed to building landfills to take care of our own waste," she says. "But we're not going to take care of someone else's waste, too."

Trash Knows No Borders

Many in the waste-disposal industry agree that it's ludicrous to send garbage rolling hundreds of miles. Trucking merely transfers waste from one state to another. At best, it's a short-term fix for getting rid of garbage. At worst, it's a waste of millions of dollars. Waste-disposal experts argue that the challenge is to shorten the long haul by fostering regional cooperation—neighboring states working together to solve the universal problem of garbage disposal. After all, garbage doesn't recognize state borders.

No matter how much waste they reduce or recycle, some towns will still have to truck the ash that's left after burning, or the garbage that can't be buried locally. And before we dump on New Jersey, we should recognize that it's the country's industrial "breadbasket." If Ohio and Indiana are going to take crepe soles and pharmaceuticals made in New Jersey, isn't it also fair that they take some of New Jersey's garbage? The problem, of course, is that they're taking too much.

Empowering states to levy a surcharge on imported waste—when federal regulators deem an exporting state lacks an environmentally sound disposal plan—may slow waste exportation. Yet until solutions are hammered out, and New York and New Jersey shoulder more of the responsibility for reducing, recycling, and siting additional disposal facilities, the trash will just keep on truckin'.

"I don't mind hauling it as long as I don't have to touch it," says trucker Tom Green as he climbs into his cab, bound from Brooklyn to Atwater, Ohio. "Once I'm on the road, no one but me knows I've got garbage on board."

Source: Bill Breen, *Garbage* (January/February 1991), pp. 48–51.

removed from sight. Despite its potential long-term consequences, ocean dumping was for many years one of the standard means used by coastal cities to dispose of solid waste, primarily because of its relatively low cost. However, its popularity has been severely damaged in recent years by increasing public awareness of ocean dumping's long-term environmental costs. Its popularity was further damaged in the late 1980s by a barrage of unfavorable publicity and newspaper headlines generated when syringes and other medical debris from errant or illegal ocean dumping repeatedly fouled many East Coast beaches during the summer season.

The modern-day alternative to the open dump is the **sanitary landfill**. The location of a properly sited sanitary landfill is carefully chosen to ensure that drainage from the site will not find its way into the local ecosystem, particularly surfacewater and groundwater supplies. On arrival at a sanitary landfill, waste is compacted by bulldozers and other heavy machinery. This is done both to save precious space and to eliminate pockets of air and liquids, whose presence can accelerate the creation of **leachate**, a soup of wastes that can ooze through the soil. Each day, a new mass of soil 15 to 30 centimeters thick is pushed over the trash to keep out rodents and vermin. But this is often a flimsy barrier to pests and to gases escaping from the decomposing garbage. In practice, the distinction between a sanitary landfill and an open dump is not always clear-cut.

Whatever their liabilities and shortcomings, sanitary landfills are exceedingly popular. Between 80 and 90 percent of all solid waste generated in this country currently finds its way to a sanitary landfill. But there are problems. All over the United States, sanitary landfills are filling up and closing down; and as they close down, they are not being replaced. Between 1984 and 1989, an estimated 30 percent of all U.S. landfills shut down. [9] Another third of the roughly 6,000 remaining landfills are expected to close by 1993. [10] One result is that an increasing volume of solid waste is being hauled cross-country for disposal, an expensive and wasteful practice. (For further information, see "Truckin' Trash" on page 91.) Clearly, landfills are not the wave of the future in solid-waste disposal. What are the alternatives?

Energy from Refuse

In an era of limits, perhaps the most promising disposal option is the one used daily by the millions of Americans who live in apartment buildings with incinerators. Cities and counties in at least 40 states are operating, building, or considering resource-

Sanitary landfill: An area of land built up from deposits of solid waste in layers covered by soil.

Leachate: A solution that results from the dissolving of soluble substances by downward-percolating groundwater.

FIGURE 5.3
A Solid Waste Energy Recovery Plant

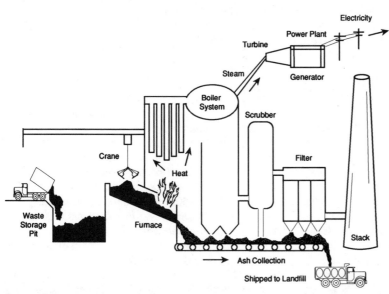

Source: Environmental Protection Agency.

Plants such as the one depicted here seek to turn a liability (solid waste) into an asset by converting it to energy. Since 80 to 90 percent of all municipal solid wastes are burnable, they can be used as a boiler fuel without resorting to costly separation. The energy generated is then sold at market prices, and the remaining residue (ash) is shipped to a landfill or other disposal site.

Did You Know That . . .

Almost 90 percent of America's trash is dumped into landfills each year, and 6 percent is burned. By contrast, Japan recycles 45 percent of its waste and disposes of 82 percent of the remainder through incineration.

recovery plants to burn their trash. The process as applied to waste disposal is more complex than simply setting fire to a mass of garbage in an open dump. In a modern waste-to-energy facility, trash is burned in a carefully engineered furnace and the heat is used to produce steam that can be sold for industrial or public use. Thus, to many officials, trash is not garbage, it is solid fuel. The methane escaping from the Fresh Kills Dump on Staten Island, yellow mounds that could be mistaken for sand dunes if it were not for the stench, could heat 50,000 houses.

One of the virtues of incineration is that it promises to turn a disposal problem into a source of energy. Most modern incineration plants are in fact designed to generate power. The difference is that they use "garbage" for fuel instead of coal, oil, or nuclear

(continued on p. 97)

The Past Imperfect Life of Incinerators

The incinerator, a device whose popularity has enjoyed enormous ups and suffered enormous downs during the hundred years since its introduction, was one of the very first of our technological fixes for garbage disposal. Before we explore that topic, however, let's look back at "reduction," a kind of cross between recycling and meltdown.

New York City's 19th-century sanitation chief, Colonel George E. Waring, Jr., was the real force behind reduction. Waring at first tried to get the general public to participate in what today would be called a "curbside separation program"—putting out the trash with glass, paper, and "wet" garbage in separate bundles—so as to recycle glass and paper. He soon gave up the idea when New Yorkers proved, to use his word, "obdurate." In 1898 Waring founded the Sanitation Utilization Company and gave recycling another try. The goal this time was "reduction," a technique imported from Europe but never widely adopted there, in which wet garbage and dead animals (Waring's White Wings sanitation force carried some 15,000 dead horses off the streets every year) were stewed in large vats in order to produce grease and a substance called residuum. The grease was sold for the manufacture of soap, candles, glycerine, lubricants, and perfume. The residuum was used for fertilizer. The Sanitation Utilization Company turned a handsome profit and reduction plants were soon in operation throughout the United States.

One reason for the success of reduction was that, by world standards, the country was rich; its garbage was surprisingly rich, too, and so were the liquids that could be distilled from it. The negative side of reduction was that the plants emitted pungent odors as well as a black, molten runoff that polluted nearby streams. Most reduction plants were shut down by the 1920s as impossibly disgusting (the last one, however, closed in 1957, in Philadelphia), leaving a vacancy that was quickly filled by incinerators.

The first garbage incinerator, known as a "de-structor," was opened in Nottingham, England, in 1874. The U.S. Army built the first American model, called a "cremator," on Governor's Island in New York City in 1885. By 1920 there were incinerators in twelve American cities, and on the eve of World War II some 700 incinerators were in operation. And then, rather abruptly, incinerators fell into a period of decline. The advantages of incinerators were always well known (they burned garbage) but so were the disadvantages (they discharged foul odors, noxious gases, and gritty smoke). For aesthetic reasons rather than reasons of health or the environment—this was before we had heard of "risk factors"—municipalities in the 1950s began shutting down their incinerators and switching to a disposal regime centered on the sanitary landfill. Within a few years of the passage of the Clean Air Act of 1970, there were only 67 incinerators still in operation in the U.S.

Then came the energy crisis, and soon afterwards an object lesson in why making policy during a crisis so often leads to undesirable results. Amid skyrocketing fuel costs and a fear of resource shortages, incinerators were reinvented, retooled, and renamed. Building a "resource-recovery plant" came to be seen almost as a patriotic duty. By 1977 some 20 new incinerators were on line, another 10 were being built, and about 35 were on the drawing board.

Yet resource-recovery plants tried to accomplish too much. A surfeit of variables had to be factored into their operations. The plants were dependent for their profitability on sales of recovered materials, but the secondary-materials markets are exceedingly erratic and in any event already serviced by a small army of professional traders. Many plants had difficulty just getting enough garbage to operate—their tipping fees were higher than those charged by landfills, or they had used generic estimates and miscalculated the quantity of refuse generated locally. Today, only a few resource-recovery plants remain in operation.

The newest means of incineration, a European import called mass burn, will have more staying power because it is simple. The main drawback is that, for all their pollution controls, these incinerators can release into the atmosphere small amounts of some 27 metals and acid gases. No one really knows what the long-term risks are.

Incinerators can usually be operated safely—for a time. But plants get old, and performance begins to decline. Nevertheless, incineration is a big piece of the future, and environmentalists—at least mainstream environmentalists—seem more-or-less resigned to mass-burn plants as the only conceivable alternative to a continuing reliance on landfills, many of which . . . are old and not located in safe places.

Source: W. L. Rathje, *Garbage* (March/April 1991), pp. 46–47.

power. Another is that incineration can be a relatively clean process from the environmental standpoint. To be sure, there are certain requirements that must be met for this to occur. It is extremely important that the solid-waste "fuel" be properly prepared by sorting. In addition, the plant must be properly equipped with pollution-control devices and be run by highly skilled and specially trained workers.

Any "plus" is bound to have a few minus points, however, and incineration is no exception. The most important, and by far the most controversial of these, has to do with the ash that is the inevitable end-product of the incineration process. Among the ingredients that make up this ash are at least 27 metals known to have potentially harmful effects on humans. Chief among these are lead, cadmium, and dioxins. The potential health effects of human exposure to these substances include kidney damage, pulmonary disease, and a host of other ills. Many of these substances are also harmful to the bacteria needed to treat sewage. Incinerator ash must, therefore, be treated with care.

So too must the basic design of the incineration plant. One of the hazards to be avoided is the excess emission of hydrogen chloride and hydrochloric acid, toxic by-products that irritate the eyes, nose, and throat and contribute to the acid-rain dilemma. The most common source of these emissions are the PVCs in packaging material. Because of this, incinerators that burn PVCs must have scrubbers to prevent emissions of hydrogen chloride and hydrochloric acid. Properly designed scrubbers can be highly effective. In contrast to an earlier study that suggested incineration plants in the United States emit more than 40 times the level of hydrogen chloride generated by coal-burning facilities, recent tests by the New York State Department of Environmental Conservation demonstrated that properly designed and operated incinerators do not emit significant quantities of either hydrochloric acid or dioxins (another by-product of burning PVCs). And, because of its chlorine content, PVC can be viewed as a worst-case example of the problems posed by incineration. [11]

Despite potential problems, incineration today ranks as the number-2 method of garbage disposal in the United States, with 128 trash-to-energy plants in operation and at least 19 more under construction. [12] Most if not all of the problems associated with incineration, save perhaps for the problem of ash disposal, currently have technical solutions. But like most such solutions, these are not cheap, prompting the need to consider other approaches to the solid-waste problem.

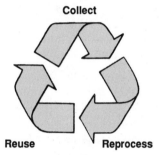

Recycling

One way to deal with the growing volume of solid wastes is to find ever more efficient and environmentally sound methods of disposal. Another is to cut the solid-waste mountain down to size by reducing the volume of material to be disposed of. One way to do this is by recycling. As landfill sites dwindle and dump fees soar, recycling has become increasingly popular with the American public. In a recent consumer survey, for example, 95 percent of those responding indicated they were willing to recycle. [13]

One of the reasons for recycling's popularity is that it increasingly makes both economic and environmental sense while simultaneously contributing to improved public health. Despite problems, both industry and consumers are learning to recycle. On the consumer front, a steadily increasing number of municipalities (and some states) have enacted mandatory recycling laws, reflecting a groundswell of popular support. And the public effort has increasingly been duplicated by businesses, sometimes with immediate, financially beneficial results. A paper-recycling program instituted by Hewlett Packard in Palo Alto, California, converted a $40,000-a-month expense for trash removal to a $2,000-a-month source of income. [14] A similar effort by AT&T, which had been spending $1 million a year getting rid of paper, generated over $365,000 in revenue in 1988. [15]

This is not to suggest that recycling always pays, at least not in the sense of generating revenue. Nonetheless, when viewed as a "disposal" option, recycling is often the most cost-effective alternative. With recycling, the real bottom line is lower taxes, energy savings, and a cleaner and more healthful environment. As one author noted, "Recycling offers communities everywhere the opportunity to trim their waste disposal needs, and thereby reduce disposal costs, while simultaneously combating global environmental problems." [16]

Selected Successful Industrial Waste Reduction Efforts

Company/Location	Products	Strategy and Efforts
Astra Södertälje, Sweden	Pharmaceuticals	Improved in-plant recycling and substitution of water for solvents cut toxic wastes by half.
Borden Chem. California, United States	Resins; adhesives	Altered rinsing and other operating procedures cut organic chemicals in wastewater by 93 percent; sludge disposal costs reduced by $49,000 per year.
Cleo Wrap Tennessee, United States	Gift wrapping paper	Substitution of water-based for solvent-based ink virtually eliminated hazardous waste, saving $35,000 per year.
Duphar Amsterdam, The Netherlands	Pesticides	New manufacturing process cut toxic waste per unit of one chemical produced from 20 kilograms to 1.
Du Pont Barranquilla, Columbia	Pesticides	New equipment to recover chemical used in making a fungicide reclaims materials valued at $50,000 annually; waste discharges were cut 95 percent.

Source: R. Caplan et al., *Our Earth, Ourselves: The Action-Oriented Guide to Help You Protect and Preserve Our Planet* (New York: Bantam Books, 1990), p. 138.

The logic of recycling has not gone unnoticed outside the United States. The Japanese, for example, have for some time been recycling more than half of their waste paper. Think about the benefits of doing this: making paper from recyclables reduces the energy used in paper production by 75 percent while saving forests, too. The high-fiber white paper increasingly used in offices is precisely the right stuff for recycling. In Japan, 95 percent of the beer bottles have been used approximately 20 times (Americans recycle only 7 percent of their glass). [17] In France, 100 local composting plants produce 800,000 tons of compost from appropriately separated garbage. As one writer puts it, "We are literally throwing away our future." [18]

While the United States is still playing ecological catch-up with many countries, Americans seem to be learning fast (sometimes, admittedly, with a little coaxing from new laws and fines). Crushed glass is being used as a filler in road surfacing, now

Americans have found a lot to admire in Japan's ability to make products. But the United States also has much to learn about how Japan *disposes* of its used products and other solid wastes, according to a report by INFORM, a nonprofit research group in New York City. With its small land area, high population density and scarce resources, Japan long ago came to grips with waste disposal problems that the United States is just now facing, say study authors.

The Japanese Do Garbage Better, Too

They found that while the Japanese put at most 20 percent of their unprocessed household wastes into landfills, Americans dump 90 percent of theirs. And unlike most U.S. dump sites, Japanese dumps use impermeable liners, leachate collectors and waste-water treatment to prevent pollutants from escaping into groundwater. Japan also greatly emphasizes recycling. For example, it recycles 50 percent of its paper, and 95 percent of its beer bottles are reused an average of 20 times. In contrast, 25 percent of U.S. paper and 7 percent of U.S. glass is recycled.

INFORM figures that after recycling, only half as much waste per person is generated in Japan as in the United States. And much of what is not recycled is incinerated in Japanese facilities that produce energy as a by-product. INFORM researchers found that the Japanese also take measures to ensure that the potentially toxic ash is insulated from groundwater, while in the United States, the Environmental Protection Agency does not regulate the disposal of incinerator ash because it has not decided how to test ash toxicity.

INFORM concludes that much of Japan's success is due to close coordination among national, regional and local governments in collecting disposal data and managing waste—a situation that does not exist in the United States.

Source: *Science News*, 2 January 1988, p. 9.

called "glasphalt." Hundreds of paper mills now use only reclaimed paper. Government contractors are required to purchase items with the highest available level of recovered material.

Smarter shopping and changes in consumption habits will help, but the lion's share of the solution to the waste problem goes to recycling. It simply makes sense on every level:

From a national perspective, recycling is attractive and deserves precedence over incineration and landfilling because it can contribute to national goals such as energy and materials

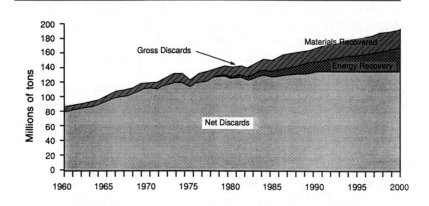

FIGURE 5.4
Recovering Solid Waste for Reuse

Solid waste can be viewed as a potential resource as well as a problem. As the above figure based on EPA projections suggests, the proportion of the solid waste stream being recovered for reuse either in the form of energy or recyled materials is increasing slowly but steadily, a trend that is expected to continue.

conservation. From a local perspective, recycling is attractive because of its potential to divert at least some materials from landfills or incinerators, which helps conserve available capacity; it also can reduce waste management costs and reduce risks to human health and the environment in some cases. [19]

TOXIC WASTES

One of the more hopeful aspects of the solid-waste problem is that much of the mountain of waste we currently throw away is composed of materials that can, in fact, be recycled or reused. The largest single component—41 percent by weight—of solid waste in the United States is paper. An additional 18 percent (by weight) is yard waste, 8.7 percent is metals, 8.2 percent is glass, 7.9 percent is food, 6.5 percent is plastics, with wood comprising an additional 3.7 percent. [20]

But buried in the stream of solids are a host of toxic substances whose presence poses health risks out of proportion to their 1 percent share of the whole. Among these are pesticides, asbestos, benzene, vinyl chloride, arsenic, and a variety of heavy metals, including chromium, cadmium, copper, and nickel. Worse, our knowledge is sadly incomplete. Of the more than 48,000 chemicals currently listed by the EPA, we know little or next to nothing about the potential toxicity of almost 38,000. [21] What we *do* know is bad enough. We know, for example, that under certain conditions, cadmium can cause kidney damage, that chromium can damage the lungs, that copper can impair the liver, and that many of the 37,000 known pesticides are extremely toxic to humans. Mounds of garbage are one thing. Although unsightly, they are at least visible. But with toxic wastes, it is often what we do not see that hurts us.

The Mechanisms of Harm

The mechanisms by which these substances harm us are various. Some, such as pesticides, are stored in the fat of human beings and animals, accumulating in body tissue, where they damage vital organs and sometimes cause death. Pesticides have played major roles in increasing food production and in controlling diseases such as malaria and yellow fever. Yet these chemicals have become a threat, too. They are easily spread through the environment, where they persist—especially, of course, in farming regions. Drinking-water supplies in such areas where 90 percent of the drinking water comes from the ground are particularly vulnerable to contamination by **leaching**. Leaching is the term for the dispersing of soluble wastes (of all types) through the soil by the liquid that forms and percolates in landfills, subsequently entering the food chain or the water we drink.

Some toxic wastes, such as asbestos, benzene, vinyl chloride, and arsenic, are **carcinogenic** (causing a range of cancers). Others are **teratogenic** (causing birth defects) or **mutagenic** (triggering mutations in genes). More frequently than we would probably like to know, substances we discard at home and in our offices come back to haunt us. Many of these substances are harmless when stored and used as directed but can release toxic fumes or particles when dumped.

We have much more to learn about toxicity levels of many harmful substances. Industry spokespersons sometimes point to the fact that laboratory tests are conducted on "worst-case" scenarios that would require extremely high exposure levels over extended periods of time to duplicate in real life.

The harmful effects of some substances, however, have been

Leaching: The process by which soluble substances found in the soil and in landfills are dissolved and carried away by groundwater.

Carcinogenic: A term used to describe any substance or agent known to cause cancer (a carcinogen).

Teratogenic: A term used to describe any substance or agent known to cause birth defects (a teratogen).

Mutagenic: A term used to describe any substance or agent known to cause or increase the rate of genetic mutation; a mutagen.

well documented. In the United States, EPA surveys in the late 1970s revealed that nearly a third of nursing mothers had measurable amounts of PCBs—poisons whose chemical structure is similar to that of the pesticide DDT—in their milk. EPA regulations now stipulate that all material containing PCBs (electrical equipment, solvents for paints and inks, plastics, for example) must be specially labeled and disposed of only at EPA-approved waste-disposal sites. Even so, PCBs illustrate the persistence of the "waste chain." Although production of these organic compounds was banned in the United States in 1979, their continuing presence, mostly in fresh water and in human body fat, makes them an ongoing health problem.

There is, as yet, no definitive solution to the problem of toxic waste. Early identification and careful handling of hazardous wastes is clearly essential to minimizing human exposure and keeping these substances out of the food chain. Beyond this, there is the problem of disposal. Here, the primary option is the so-called "secure" landfill. One of these, in Pinewood, South Carolina, accepts about 135,000 tons of toxic waste annually. It is modern, well engineered, scrupulously clean—and hated by area residents. Nonetheless, Pinewood represents a giant step forward from the way in which toxic waste was handled at Love Canal in upstate New York.

Love Canal: A Toxic Waste Disaster

Until the late 1970s, the name "Love Canal" referred simply to a pleasant neighborhood near the industrial town of Niagara Falls, New York. The area took its name from William T. Love, an entrepreneur who in the late 19th century attempted unsuccessfully to build a canal, only to end up in bankruptcy. After World War II, the area was acquired by the Hooker Chemical and Plastics Corporation, which, between 1947 and 1952, dumped approximately 21,800 tons of pesticides, cleaning solutions, and other toxic wastes into the canal. In 1953 Hooker covered the site with dirt and sold it to the Niagara Falls Board of Education for $1. The board—which had signed papers stipulating that it would not hold Hooker responsible for any injuries or deaths that might occur—then built a school on the site, in the process puncturing the cap Hooker had installed over the landfill. The board then sold adjoining property to real-estate developers, who erected housing. Families soon settled in the area.

In 1978 heavy rains and snowfalls caused the canal to overflow, spilling its contents. Chemicals such as benzene, PCBs, and C-56 (a by-product of the manufacture of pesticides that can

(continued on p. 106)

27 Ways to Beat the Garbage Crisis

The following suggestions are based on the most successful recycling programs in the U.S. and abroad. Some may not apply to your particular situation. Select those that do. You'll be surprised how much you save—things, materials, and money—and how satisfying it is to take part in the process of reducing waste and helping clean up and prevent environmental pollution.

1. *Recycle at home and at work.* Separate newspapers (in bundles), bottles, and cans for delivery to (or pickup by) your local recycling unit. If you don't have one, see tip 24 below.

2. *Use paper scraps* for notes and memos. Reuse manila envelopes by putting on new labels (this was done widely in World War II).

3. *Reduce junk mail* by writing to the Direct Marketing Association, 6 East 43rd Street, New York, NY 10017, and asking to be taken off mailing lists. This will reduce unsolicited mail by 75 percent but will not affect mail from companies that already have your name and address. To control the latter you can send the mail back to its originator by circling the return address with a felt pen and having your name taken off mailing lists of publications you don't want.

4. *Complain* to companies that have started to package their periodicals and other products in plastic; include the wrapper in your letter. Persuade them to use wrappers made of 100 percent plant-fiber cellulose, which are more transparent than most plastics. For more information on this and on other recycled paper products contact Conservatree Paper Company at (800) 522-9200 or in California, (415) 433-1000.

5. *Buy products packaged in glass, paper, or metal containers.* Where possible, avoid aluminum (unless it is recycled) because it requires huge amounts of energy to produce. It is also thought by some researchers to be associated with Alzheimer's disease. For food, glass is safest, compared with plastics, which may diffuse to the liquids they hold, or paper products, which may contain trace amounts of dioxin.

6. *Reuse glass containers* for storing flour, rice, oatmeal, nuts, grains, and staples you can buy in bulk to save unnecessary packaging and money. They are also handy for pencils, pens, paper clips, pushpins, screws, and other household or office items.

7. *Shop where you find produce without plastic wrapping,* preferably organically grown and sold at local farmers' markets.

8. *Take along your own shopping bag,* as do consumers in other parts of the world and have it packed with groceries and other purchases. String bags are very good for this purpose. Be careful, however, that you don't get accused of shoplifting! Some supermarkets now charge for plastic bags or give discounts to customers who bring in their own bags. Encourage your local managers to adopt a similar policy.

9. *If you must choose between paper and plastic products, the better choice depends on where you live.* If they are likely to get into the ocean or lake, use paper. If you live away from water, some plastics are preferable, *with the major exception of PVCs (polyvinyl chlorides), styrofoam, and PET plastics, which are highly toxic in their manufacture and when incinerated.* Polyethylene, the very thin plastic used for bags, baggies, and translucent products such as cups and "glasses," is less polluting than paper on a per pound basis.

10. *Invest in durables.* A leather bag may cost more than a plastic one, but will outlive it by five or six times. The same principle applies to appliances, machinery, automobiles, and toys. Remember those great products from the 1950s and before—Waring blenders (mine goes back to 1947 and still works), Parker fountain pens, and Singer sewing machines. Many are still manufactured, while others you can find secondhand or discarded at recycling centers.

11. *Be an informed buyer.* Check carefully with *Consumer Reports* and other independent consumer guides before making major purchases so that you buy durable products. . . .

12. *Use cloth diapers,* if you have a baby, instead of plastic ones that dump an estimated 2.8 million tons of feces and urine into our overcrowded landfills and spread harmful bacteria. If you don't want to wash diapers, find a rental service or persuade one to serve your area. They are at least 20 percent cheaper than buying plastic diapers. For further information contact the *National Association of Diaper Services,* 2017 Walnut Street, Philadelphia, PA 19103, who will help you find a local cloth diaper service.

13. *Take a china coffee mug or teacup and metal spoon to work* so that you don't have to use tacky plastic cups and stirrers. This usually gets you more coffee or tea, is more enjoyable to use, and cuts down on waste.

14. *Avoid styrofoam.* For picnics and cookouts, wash and reuse heavy paper plates and plastic spoons and forks instead of lightweight styrofoam. If you do a lot of outdoor entertaining, consider metal camping pots and utensils, available at camping supply stores.

15. *Compost your food and other organic wastes* (leaves, grass clippings) for your garden, if you have a backyard. If you live in an apartment, propose to your neighbors to have the entire building's organic garbage sent to a local composting center.

16. *Use scrap paper and cardboard packaging as fire starters,* if you have a wood-burning stove.

17. *Reuse materials to make things you need:* old sheets, curtains, or clothes can be cut into small pieces for rags or made into hooked rugs or quilts (a few years ago I made camera lens protectors out of a 10-year-old wool shirt that had seen better days). Old lumber can be used in small home-carpentry projects or, if it is not painted or pressure-treated, as firewood (I salvage lumber and other building materials from construction sites, dumpsters, and—with permission—from our local landfill); old bricks and broken concrete make good retaining walls, garden walkways, or patios. Large (2-liter) plastic soda bottles make wonderful mini-greenhouses for growing seeds and plants: all you need is a utility knife or a pair of scissors to separate the bottle into two parts; punch holes in the bottom and use for germinating seeds; the top half works well as a solar dome to put over the plants when they have grown to about two inches. This method will save you money and give you a jump of 3 to 4 weeks on the growing season.

18. *Rent or borrow items you use infrequently—*specialized power tools, ladders, or audiovisual equipment, for example.

19. *Maintain and repair* appliances, tools, and other equipment to lengthen their lives.

20. *Share, barter, trade, or donate* what you no longer need, but which has value to others—magazines, books, toys, clothes, and other items. Thrift shops are excellent places to find what you want and to give what you don't need. You often can get a better tax deduction by donating equipment to a nonprofit group such as Greenpeace or your local Sierra Club chapter rather than by trying to resell it.

21. *Have a garage sale or charity drop-off* instead of trashing household goods.

22. *Get children interested* in making things out of newspaper, toilet paper rolls, ice-cream sticks and other throwaways. You can't be too young to get the recycling "bug."

23. *Support the national campaign to boycott styrofoam and limit the use of plastics.* Vermont and Maine have already banned state use of plastic packages. Suffolk County, N.Y. has banned plastic grocery bags and plastic food containers. Santa Monica, Calif., has banned styrofoam at two McDonald's and is considering a citywide prohibition of styrofoam cups. . . . [Ed. McDonald's abandoned the use of styrofoam packaging nationwide in late 1990.]

24. *Support recycling projects in your community.* If there isn't one, consider getting a group together. Talk to neighbors and at social gatherings. Speak up at PTA and town meetings. Write to your local newspaper explaining the advantages of recycling. Ask at your local food co-op. If you have a modem, put a notice on your computer bulletin board. If not, leave a note at your local supermarket. With the help of organizations like the Environmental Action Coalition, U.S. PIRG, Greenpeace, EDF, [and similar environmentalist groups], you can find out how to get a recycling center started in your area.

25. *Contact local officials,* your mayor or first

selectperson, and your local sanitation department to voice support for far-reaching recycling and waste reductive programs to save landfill space and avoid the need for expensive and hazardous burn plants. If you can't get through by telephone, write letters or postcards, or send telegrams. Most local officials respond to hearing from their constituents, and complain they don't hear enough. Ask them where they stand on recycling. Follow up to keep the issue alive. Thank them when they do take action of which you approve.

26. *Contact state and federal officials.* Write to your state senator and assemblyperson, and to your national senators and congresspeople, to ask them what legislative action is being taken to encourage recycling. Enlist their support for ecologically sound recycling and waste reduction programs as mandated by the law.

27. *Share your recycling experience with others.* If you carry out half of the suggestions listed above, you will already be practicing Positive Ecology!

Source: J. Naar, *Design for a Livable Planet: How You Can Help Clean Up the Environment* (New York: HarperCollins, 1990), pp. 26–28.

cause damage to virtually every organ in the body) were carried by creeks into the neighborhood. Reports began to circulate of noxious odors permeating homes, of slime oozing into basements, of children coming home with painful rashes and watering eyes after swimming in a pond on the canal site. Most alarming of all were the unusually high rates of miscarriages, birth defects, liver ailments, nervous disorders, epilepsy-like seizures, genetic damage, and cancers.

Finally, the landfill's topsoil began to wash away, revealing Hooker's by-then corroded and leaking metal casks and alerting EPA officials to the disaster. Analysis revealed that the dump contained more than 80 different chemicals, including highly dangerous pesticides, solvents that damage the heart and liver, and at least 10 potential carcinogens. In addition to their physical ailments, many residents suffered considerable psychological damage.

The incident prompted federal intervention. President Jimmy Carter declared a state of emergency in the area, and 237 families were evacuated with the help of federal funds in August 1978. Many of those who were left behind, convinced that they too were in danger, joined together to take action, forming the Love Canal Homeowners' Association. Angry and frustrated, they took their case to whoever would listen: the press, local governments, the state, and even to Washington, D.C. Finally, in May 1980, President Carter responded to their pleas. He empowered the state and the EPA to relocate 710 families temporarily while the chemical quagmire was drained and the area made safe for habitation. Untold damage had been done by the time the government took action; nevertheless, the Love Canal homeowners, who were powerless individuals when they started out, demonstrated that a well-organized, determined group *can* prod a slow-moving government into taking action on their behalf. Now, over a decade later, Love Canal is once again ready for occupancy.

Much remains to be done, however. The EPA has identified at least 29,000 additional toxic waste sites that require cleanup, while some have estimated that there may be as many as 290,000 locations in this country where toxic wastes threaten underground sources of drinking water. Nor is the problem of toxic waste restricted to the United States. From industrial landfills in Germany to overloaded sewage systems in India to the noxious chemical soup that poisons so many Eastern European water sources, toxic wastes pose a global threat to human health. No country and no person is immune.

Taking Steps Toward a Healthier Environment

TODAY THERE IS a growing awareness that all of the natural world's processes and cycles are closely related. As we have seen, the conditions that contribute to the continued good health and survival of all species, including our own, are the result of a complex balance. As we have also seen, population growth, energy use and misuse, air and water pollution, and the garbage and waste crises can upset that balance; they are all parts of a whole. As parts of that whole, each of us has a potential impact on the environment. The good news is that we can do much to undo the damage that has been done. Acting both individually and together, we can restore the balance needed for our own wellness and the survival of our species—if we act responsibly and without delay.

It is important that we act promptly. Recent books, articles, and television programs have provided scenarios of what will happen if we follow our present patterns. One of the more pessimistic of these paints the following picture of events by the year 2050:

> Global warming means rapid change, and rapid change means the end of familiar places. It means the trees that we walk among, that our forebears walked among, that we wanted our children to know, will vanish. It means that the creatures of Yellowstone will scatter and the languid salt marsh, with its clams and ducks and egrets, will be drowned. Our favorite beach will disappear and our prized trout stream will run dry. In short, it means that nature can no longer be protected and preserved, no matter how hard we try.

FIGURE 6.1
The Future of Global Oil Consumption

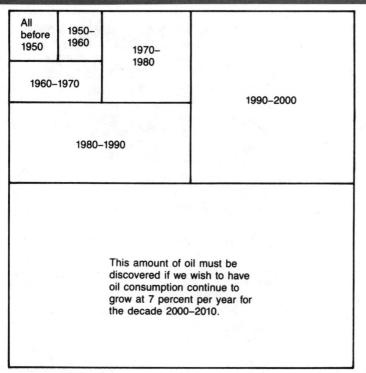

Source: Adapted from A. A. Bartlett, "Forgotten Fundamentals of the Energy Crisis," *American Journal of Physics,* 46 (1978), p. 880.

How much oil will we consume in each decade if oil consumption continues to grow at its historical rate of 7 percent a year? As much oil as has been consumed in all of previous history.

It means the air, filled with the smoke of a thousand fires, will be grayer, summer days hotter, estuaries slimier. Sunbelters will move back north, Midwesterners will move to Canada, Bangladeshis will have nowhere to go. [1]

Its author hastens to outline the ways we can achieve another, very possible outcome. The fact that nations are regularly convening to explore steps needed to preserve the global village's environment is an encouraging sign. So too are the major solar-

(continued on p. 111)

FIGURE 6.2
Energy Use per Capita for Selected Countries, 1988

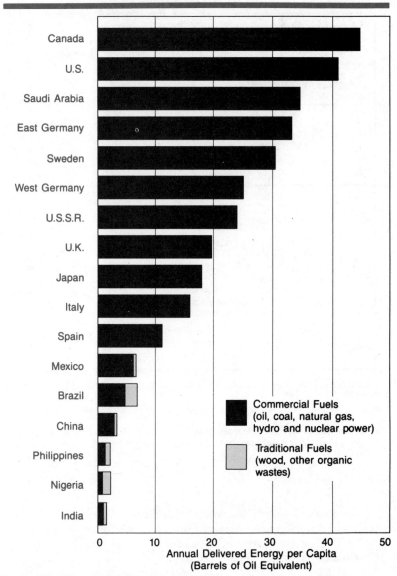

Source: *Scientific American,* September 1990, p. 57.

Great disparities exist in per capita energy use. The average citizen in the U.S. and Canada used over 40 barrels of oil in 1988. It is estimated that the U.S. could save $220 billion a year if it became as energy efficient as Japan or the United Kingdom.

energy research and development programs now under way in several nations. Unfortunately, this is an area in which the United States continues to drag its heels. In 1990 the federal budget included $44 *billion* for armed-forces research and development and only $191 *million* for all aspects of the global environment.

Whether the solutions will come via new technologies or through a new environmental ethic, some progress *is* being made. The smog problem in Los Angeles, for example, has not been solved by the use of emission-control devices in automobiles. Therefore, Los Angeles will probably be the first city to require use of nonpolluting cars. The city's plan is to reduce noxious emissions from all sources and clean up the air by 80 to 90 percent by the year 2007. Gasoline-powered vehicles will probably have to be banned. Electric- or methane-powered vehicles would be the only ones permitted in the city. Aerosol sprays, outdoor barbecues, and gasoline-powered machinery, such as lawnmowers, are also targeted by city planners. [2] Clearly, changes of this magnitude require changes of life-style as well. The technology behind more fuel-efficient automobiles or alternatives to harmful products is constantly being advanced. But the key to using these technologies is an understanding of the consequences of human activity. Learning to protect the environment so that it will protect us involves changes of attitude, changes of habit, and changes in legislation and political systems.

Did You Know That . . .

The average automobile uses approximately 15 percent more fuel at 60 miles per hour than at 50 miles per hour.

WHAT WE CAN DO INDIVIDUALLY

Individuals on this planet have in some way or another an obligation to preserve our environment for future generations. One of the most effective ways to show immediate results would be to become better informed of the complexities of our total environmental system. Reading and reflecting on the chapters of this book could be a step. Adopting plans of action to tackle the specific problems presented in each chapter—energy conservation, recycling, sensible consumerism, and so on—is another.

Changing Attitudes

The ecological "fix" we have gotten ourselves into is in large part due to the tendency to think that when it comes to the environment, tomorrow is soon enough to make changes. If we continue to believe that *someone else* will take care of things, we have given up our basic right to control our lives. Until and unless we as individuals are willing to change our ways, we cannot expect society to be concerned about environmental preservation. Without new attitudes, Madison Avenue will continue to push new products that "everyone needs" to "keep up with the Joneses." Fortunately, manufacturers and advertisers have begun to listen more attentively to those who *do* care—and the results range from unbleached-paper coffee filters (which thus avoid dioxin-laced coffee) to more environmentally considerate packaging. This was the scene in one supermarket in a suburb of New York City late in 1990:

> Ruth Stumacher was minding her own business, doing her weekly shopping at the Gristede's here when she was caught redhanded.
>
> No, her fingers hadn't dipped into the bin of chocolate-covered almonds. Her offense was graver: she had piled in her cart a few packs of juice boxes, each with its own straw, and all wrapped in plastic.
>
> "These containers are terribly overpackaged and aren't easily recycled," Mrs. Stumacher was warned by Roberta Wiernik, a League of Women Voters member leading an "environmental shopping" tour down the aisle. The handful of women taking the tour nodded knowingly; Mrs. Stumacher, who is 66 years old, put the juice boxes back.
>
> As garbage-disposal problems grow across the metropolitan region and much of the country, a new campaign is under way to persuade people not to produce so much trash in the first place. [3]

In towns across the United States, a new concept—*precycling*—has taken hold. The director of the solid-waste division of the New York State Department of Environmental Conservation puts it this way: "What we're really talking about is a societal change from our immediate-gratification, throwaway mentality to a greater awareness of the consequences." To help educate intelligent consumers, several states have adopted regulations authorizing manufacturers to use certain labels to announce products as "recycled," "reusable," or "recyclable." [4]

Reeducation of tastes and expectations is also important. Nowhere is this more true than in our role as consumers. The American consumer in particular tends to place great value on appearance and convenience and relatively little on environmental costs (which, to be fair, are often invisible or hidden). For example, it is one thing to produce and sell nutritious apples; it is another to produce and sell "perfect" apples, of uniform size and texture and wholly without blemish. To produce such apples

FIGURE 6.3
Environmentally Friendly Packaging

Did You Know That . . .

The printed design and lettering on most plastic bread wrappers contain lead.

A note on our packaging material.
Most mail order companies use plastic foam "peanuts" to fill shipping cartons. We don't. The chemicals used in their production contribute to ozone depletion and even if they didn't, peanuts don't degrade for a thousand years. In short, they are a nuisance. Instead, we cushion your orders with shredded recycled paper and in some cases - real popcorn. In addition, for every tree we use through the printing needs of our catalog our company plants two more in a program of habitat restoration.
It seems the overwhelmingly sensible thing to do - replace what you use and try and leave the world a little better than you found it.

S M I T H & H A W K E N

Socially responsible companies such as the gardening and clothing supplier, Smith and Hawken, are using more recycled products and environmentally considerate materials for packaging.

requires extensive use of chemicals and pesticides to control "bad" insects. Unfortunately, most of the chemicals used for these purposes also kill the "good" insects needed for pollination. The environmental costs of the quest for perfect apples often include a reduction in the number of beneficial insects and an overdose of pesticides—pesticides that in due course find their way into our drinking water.

The statistics are stark. There are 60 different cancer-causing substances used on fruit. [5] At the same time, 80 percent of all cancers are believed to have an environmental cause. And the consumer issue is clear. Why do we have to have perfect apples? Why can we not accept an apple with less eye appeal but just as much nutrition?

So besides education and reeducation, there must be re-

FIGURE 6.4
Reclaiming Aluminum Cans

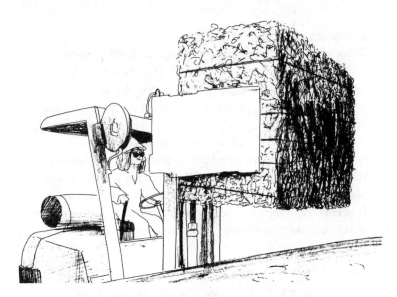

Source: Aluminum Company of America.

These 1,200-pound bales of used aluminum beverage and food cans at a reclamation mill at Alcoa, Tennessee, represent part of the more than 700 million pounds of used containers collected in 1990 by Alcoa's national recycling network. The used cans will be remelted, rolled into new can sheet and sold to can makers, closing the loop between used cans and new cans in less than 90 days. In 1990, more than 6 of every 10 aluminum beverage cans sold were recycled into new cans. Recycling aluminum cans saves energy, fights litter, and eases the burden on municipal landfills.

evaluation. As this reevaluation occurs, we will experience a "biotic reorganization." This means that we as a society will experience a shift in certain basic priorities as we become more acutely sensitive to the state of and the needs of the environment. For such a change to occur, the following conditions must be present:

1. People must want to help preserve the environment. The motivation for this must come from within. There must come a realization that *we* are the ultimate endangered species.

2. This awareness must be sufficiently widespread and powerful to prompt permanent life-style changes.

3. Efforts to control population growth must be taken out of the religious realm and evaluated within the context of the global environmental crisis.

4. Organized efforts to deal with the greenhouse effect and the depletion of the ozone layer must be given priority.

5. We must reevaluate our production of solid waste and find ways to decrease its volume.

6. We should undertake further research on how to increase our environmental awareness and appreciation for environmental values.

Everyday Actions

If such goals seem lofty or beyond our capabilities, there are more immediate steps upon which we can focus as we shop, clean, consume, and discard. Being careful about what we use, and how, will not only help the environment but will be the single most significant thing we can do to ensure our own wellness. Experts point out there has been a disproportionate amount of research and attention given to outdoor air pollution: "Even if leaking in large amounts, the chemicals from dump sites must travel through a series of environmental pathways with many chances for degradation or diversion before causing exposure. The same chemical in a can of spray paint used in the family room has a direct, fast route into the body." [6] When it comes to individual wellness or environmental harm, prevention is the wiser route. But there are means of "detoxing" our bodies and our planet.

Opportunities for improving our environment abound. We know that pure water is not plentiful. Did you know that you can reduce your use of water for showering by 27 percent? For example, a quick wet-down, soap-up, rinse-off shower consumes an average of 4 gallons, compared with a regular shower's 25. Filling a basin for shaving takes 1 gallon; leaving the tap running can use 20. [7] We know that increased levels of carbon dioxide are harmful in many ways. Did you know that planting 3 trees around your home will not only reduce the carbon dioxide and increase the oxygen level but reduce your air-conditioning costs by 10 to 50 percent? [8] The city of Los Angeles recognized this and in early 1989 announced a program of providing shade trees for homes. Similarly, the Agricultural Department's Conser-

(continued on p. 119)

Did You Know That . . .

While plastic is generally viewed as less desirable than paper from an environmental standpoint, manufacturing a paper cup uses 6 times more steam, 24 times more electricity, and produces 200 times more waste water than manufacturing a polystyrene cup.

Chemical Hazards in the Home

When you think of chemical hazards, you may think of Bhopal or the Love Canal. But these isolated industrial cases represent more immediate problems that affect you daily. Hazardous chemicals are present in virtually every American home—they're in your cleanser, your disinfectants, even the motor oil in your garage.

Hazardous household chemicals can be grouped into four categories:

Reactive products contain unstable compounds that may react with air, water, or other chemicals with dangerous results. One example is calcium hypochlorite, a powder used to disinfect swimming pools, which can react with paint or kerosene to produce explosive and toxic chlorine gas.

Corrosives are strong acids or bases that eat away other substances. Examples include chlorine bleach, a powerful acid, and drain opener, a powerful base. Corrosives can cause severe burns on contact, and their vapors can burn the eyes. They are also poisonous if ingested.

Ignitable products, like gasoline and furniture polish, pose a fire hazard if improperly stored or used.

Toxic products have perhaps the greatest

Chemical Hazards in the Home

Product	Possible Hazards	Disposal Suggestions	Precautions and Substitutes
Aerosols	When sprayed, contents are broken into particles small enough to be inhaled. Cans may explode or burn.	Put **only** empty cans in trash. Do not burn. Do not place in trash compactor.	Store in cool place. Propellant may be flammable. Instead: use non-aerosol products.
Drain cleaners	Very corrosive. May be fatal if swallowed. Contact with eyes can cause blindness.	Use up according to label instructions.	Prevention best; keep sink strainers in good condition. Instead: use plunger, plumber's snake, vinegar & baking soda followed by boiling water.
Flea powders, sprays & shampoos	Moderately to very poisonous. *Toxicity 2–4˙*	Use up or save for hazardous waste collection day.	DO NOT USE DOG PRODUCTS ON CATS Vacuum house regularly & thoroughly. Launder pet bedding frequently.
Oven cleaner	Corrosive. Very harmful if swallowed. Irritating vapors. Can cause eye damage. *Toxicity 2–4˙*	Use up according to label instructions or give away. Save for hazardous waste collection day.	Do not use aerosols, which can explode and are difficult to control. Instead: use paste. Or heat oven to 200 degrees, turn off, leave small dish of ammonia in oven overnight, then wipe oven with damp cloth and baking soda. Do not put baking soda on heating elements.
Toilet bowl cleaner	Corrosive. May be fatal if swallowed. *Toxicity 3–4˙*	Use up according to label instructions or wash down the sink or toilet with lots of water.	Ventilate room. Instead: use ordinary cleanser or detergent and baking soda.

Chemical Hazards in the Garage and Workshop

Product	Possible Hazards	Disposal Suggestions	Precautions and Substitutes
Aerosols	When sprayed, contents are broken into particles small enough to be inhaled. Cans may explode or burn.	Put **only** empty cans in trash. Do not burn. Do not place in trash compactor.	Store in cool place. Propellant may be flammable. Instead: use non-aerosol products.
Auto: antifreeze	Very poisonous. Has sweet taste—attractive to small children & pets. *Toxicity 3–4`*`	Amounts of less than 1 gallon pour down sink with plenty of water. Do **not** do this if you have a septic tank. Put in a secure container & take to a garage or service station.	No substitutes. Clean up any leaks or spills carefully.
Auto: batteries	Contain strong acid. Very corrosive. Danger to eyes & skin.	Recycle.	No substitutes. Trade in old batteries.
Auto: degreasers	Corrosive. Poisonous. Eye & skin irritant. *Toxicity 2–4`*`	Use up according to label instructions.	Choose strong detergent type over solvent type.
Auto: motor oil & transmission fluid	Poisonous. May be contaminated with lead. Skin & eye irritant.	Recycle.	No substitutes.
Paint strippers, thinners, & other solvents	Many are flammable. Eye & skin irritant. Moderately to very poisonous. *Toxicity 3–4`*`	Let settle, pour off cleaner for re-use. Pour sludge into container & seal, or wrap well in newspaper & throw in trash. Use up according to label instructions or save for hazardous waste collection day.	Avoid aerosols. Buy only as much as you need. Ventilate area well. Do not use near open flame. Instead of paint stripper: sand or use heat gun. Use water cleanup products as much as possible.
Paints, oil-based, & varnishes	Flammable. Eye & skin irritant. Use in small, closed area may cause unconsciousness.	Use up according to label instructions or save for hazardous waste collection day.	Ventilate area well. Do not use near open flame. May take weeks for fumes to go away. Instead: use water-based paints if possible.
Pesticides`**`, herbicides, fungicides, slugbait, rodent poison, wood preservatives	All are dangerous to some degree. Can cause central nervous system damage, kidney & liver damage, birth defects, internal bleeding, eye injury. Some are readily absorbed through the skin. *Toxicity 3–6`*`	Use up carefully, following label instructions. Save for hazardous waste collection day.	Do not buy more than you need. Instead: try hand-picking, mechanical cultivation, natural predators. Practice good sanitation. Choose hardy varieties. Use insect lures & traps. As a last resort, use least toxic suitable pesticides.

*General Toxicity Rating

Number Rating	1	2	3	4	5	6
Toxicity Rating	Almost Non-Toxic	Slightly Toxic	Moderately Toxic	Very Toxic	Extremely Toxic	Super Toxic
Lethal Dose for 150 lb. Adult	More than 1 Quart	1 Pint to 1 Quart	1 Ounce to 1 Pint	1 Teaspoon to 1 Ounce	7 Drops to 1 Teaspoon	Less Than 7 Drops

For more information, contact your local public works department, hazardous waste agency, or poison control center.

**The following pesticides previously sold for use by homeowners and the general public have since been banned, or are no longer recommended for use by homeowners:

- Aldrin
- Arsenate
- Calcium Arsenate
- Chlordane

- Copper Arsenate
- Creosote
- DDT
- Dieldrin
- Heptachlor

- Pentachlorophenol (PCP)
- Silvex
- Sodium Arsenite
- 2–4–5T

If you have any of these pesticides, carefully store and save them for a hazardous waste collection day. Get a plastic container with a lid. (A five-gallon plastic bucket is ideal.) Fill the bucket halfway with cat litter. Keep the pesticide in its original container and put it in the bucket. Fill the bucket to the top with cat litter. Put the lid on it. Mark the container clearly, and store it on a shelf away from children and pets.

potential for devastation, because in addition to poisoning individual users, they can pollute the environment if improperly disposed of—in effect, poisoning the entire planet. Toxic products include herbicides and insecticides.

Many household products have multiple potential for damage; that is, they fit into more than one of the foregoing categories. Aerosols, for instance, can explode if improperly disposed of. They also disperse sometimes dangerous substances into particles small enough to be inhaled. And some chemicals in aerosol propellants destroy the earth's ozone layer.

Obviously, we need many hazardous substances in our everyday lives. But safe substitutes are available for many harmful household chemicals. Baking soda, for example, can be substituted for many harmful kitchen and bathroom cleansers.

Unfortunately, no safe substitutes exist for certain hazardous substances. In these cases, safe use and disposal practices, including recycling, can minimize the dangers such chemicals pose to you and the environment.

The National Safety Council urges you to con-sider the health and safety of yourself, your community, and the environment every time you use a hazardous household substance. Be a smart consumer. Read product labels to find out how dangerous a substance is. If you can find a nonhazardous substitute for a hazardous product, do so. Otherwise, buy only the amount you need and then use it up or give the excess to someone who can use it.

Recycle as many harmful substances as possible. If you can't recycle, be sure to follow proper disposal procedures. Improper disposal of hazardous chemicals can injure trash collectors, other waste management personnel, and the environment. After solid garbage is collected, it is sent to municipal landfills. Eventually, chemicals in landfills can erode protective liners and enter the local groundwater. Certain liquid chemicals cannot be adequately treated by wastewater facilities. Liquid chemicals that end up in septic tanks often seep through and contaminate local groundwater. Throwing some hazardous substances into the trash or down the drain can have a devastating effect on lakes, rivers, and drinking water supplies. If you need to dispose of a hazardous chemical in your home, and the product label does not give disposal advice, call your local public health or sanitation department. They will explain how to dispose of the substance, or tell you when your community's next hazardous waste collection day will be.

Modern technology has brought us many advances but, in the process, it also has brought us to a threshold of danger. The chemical substances we have come to rely on for our existence may be the agents of our destruction. Proper use of these substances is our responsibility. Our future, as individuals and as a global community, depends on it.

Source: *Healthline*, February 1990, pp. 11–13.

vation Reserve now pays farmers to plant trees on land that is subject to erosion. [9]

These are but a few examples of the many small but positive steps each of us can take as individuals. The main thing to remember is: taken together, our individual actions will help create a healthier environment.

THE BIGGER PICTURE AND YOU

Of course, many environmental problems cannot be adequately addressed without the direction or intervention of local, state, national, or international governmental bodies. You still can make a difference through advocacy. In fact, it is sometimes essential that you do so. A national public-policy group called Renew America, which ranks state and local efforts at environmental protection, termed the deterioration of the total environment over the past 25 years as "business-as-usual pollution." The problems have been exacerbated by budget cuts and policy decisions that shift environmental-protection activities from the federal government to the states at a time when state budgets are already struggling with the costs of coping with social problems, such as education, drugs, and crime.

The fact that air pollution and acid rain cause adverse effects on human health, resulting in lost workdays because people suffer more respiratory diseases, and that this ongoing cost exceeds the price of emissions controls; that air pollution and acid rain kill life in vulnerable lakes, streams, estuaries, and forests, natural-resource bases that may take centuries to recover; that they cause the corrosion of bridges, buildings, and monuments; and that they hasten the destruction of books and works of art that are the highest expressions of human thought and cre-

FIGURE 6.5

Energy Guide for Major Appliances

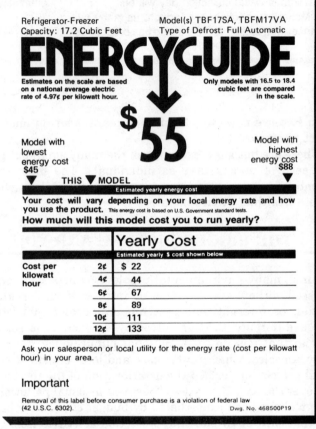

The energy guide depicted here is now attached to most major appliances. Buying a more energy-efficient unit may be more expensive initially, but could save you money over the lifetime of the appliance.

ativity—all of this counts for naught to most members of Congress, who pantingly ask the really *big* question: "*What's in it for my district?*" In the real world, the key to solving big problems is that each individual constituency must see its own particular advantage in the larger solution. [10]

Some of the handbooks cited in the appendix provide suggestions—even form letters—to assist you in making your particular concerns heard. Look to your own community too. Local branches of The Nature Conservancy, for example, have done much to preserve green space, countless species, and resources that are vital to the ecological balance. Citizen groups have spearheaded recycling efforts. In some states, such as California, for example, public conservation corps have helped to build parks, save energy by updating lighting and heating, and plant trees. Pressure groups have persuaded manufacturers to improve their packaging. It was a grass-roots movement that led to the EPA ban on the use of CFCs in aerosol cans. Environmentalists are currently pushing Congress to regulate smaller industrial polluters under the Clean Water Act. Neighborhoods have banded together and caused groups like the Chemical Industry Council of Maryland to become "born-again environmentalists."

As people left the land to adopt urban life-styles and demanded more and more sophisticated technologies, they left the judgments about the wisdom of those technologies to "others." It is time to get back in touch with the land and to reclaim control or at least, as one observer remarked, learn "how to worry together as a species [which] may well be our next essential evolutionary turning point." [11]

A PLAN FOR ACTION

We can summarize the intent and the direction of the many specific suggestions made in this book, and others, in the following guiding principles:

1. Inform yourself and ask questions. Follow news of local as well as national and global environmental problems and identify areas where you can make a difference by altering your personal habits or participating in joint efforts.

2. Review your shopping, consumption, and disposal patterns. Do not be overwhelmed by the extent of an environmental problem but value the importance of your efforts to combat it. Look for natural ingredients in all types of products. Study ways to make your home less potentially toxic. Monitor water use and have a utility company do an energy-saving check. Recycle—and precycle—by ecologically smart shopping. Look for ways to recycle items around your house, such as reusing

(continued on p. 123)

Things You Can Do to Help the Environment

RECYCLE, REDUCE WASTE, BUY WISELY

- Buy only what you need.
- Buy products in bulk or with as little packaging as possible.
- Buy stationery and computer paper made from recycled paper.
- Buy things of wood, glass, or paper rather than plastic or styrofoam.
- Buy beverages in returnable bottles.
- Don't buy aerosol cans (CFCs destroy the ozone).
- Use phosphate-free, biodegradable soaps and detergents and non-toxic cleaning products.
- Use plates, mugs, cloth napkins, and dish towels instead of paper plates, cups, napkins, and towels.
- Use cloth diapers for infants rather than disposables.
- Avoid fast food restaurants, with their excessive use of styrofoam, plastic, and paper packaging.
- Recycle motor oil, glass bottles, cans, cardboard, office paper, plastic, and newspaper.
- Don't buy tropical wood, unless you are sure it is from a sustainable tree farm.
- Buy locally grown produce grown without pesticides and chemical fertilizers.
- Buy at local farmers' markets.

IN THE HOME

- Have an energy audit of your home done; insulate windows, walls, attic, and water heater.
- Turn down the thermostat in winter and put on a sweater.
- Limit use of air-conditioning in home and car.
- Install water-saving shower heads, faucets, and toilet devices.
- Don't let unneeded water run while brushing teeth, or washing dishes and clothes.
- Grow a vegetable garden rather than a lawn to reduce water waste.
- Eat lower on the food chain (more grains, fruit, and vegetables; less meat).
- Hand-wash rather than have clothes dry-cleaned (dry-cleaning solvents destroy the ozone).

ON THE MOVE

- Car pool to work, walk, or ride a bike.
- Use buses and other public transportation.
- Drive a fuel-efficient car.

GET INVOLVED

- Join local environmental and neighborhood groups working on issues that affect your community.
- Lobby your city to start programs in curbside, oil, and CFC (from old refrigerators and air-conditioners) recycling.
- Pressure fast food chains to reduce use of packaging.
- Write congressmen and senators in support of timber practice reform on public lands and saving of old-growth forests.
- Support and write governmental leaders regarding agriculture reforms that encourage sustainable growing methods, small farms, organic farming practices.
- Lobby governmental leaders in support of building light rail lines, improving bus or other transportation lines in your vicinity.
- Write letters to your local newspapers on issues you are concerned about.

Source: Judith Hurley and Richard Schlaadt, *Wellness: The Wellness Life-Style* (Guilford, CT: The Dushkin Publishing Group, 1992), p. 100.

paper goods or cutting up old cloth towels for wiping up instead of using extra paper towels. Read labels and advocate more complete labeling. Dispose of hazardous products properly.

3. Maintain your own body's health by a balanced diet and supplements selected with the advice of your doctor. Look for ways to reduce the stress on your *inner* environment.

4. Speak up. Complain to manufacturers about products or production practices that pollute or endanger the planet or you. Attend local civic and regional planning boards or write legislators about concerns regarding water, air, wastes, population density, and related problems. Vote for those who you feel can be instrumental in improving the environment. Use right-to-know laws to find out if there are environmental regulation compliance problems in your community.

5. Study the efforts of various environment-action groups and decide which may be the one or 2 that you would like to support.

6. Think globally. Remember how all the species and all the nations of the Earth are connected and—through joining with others, contacting your governmental representatives, and supporting UNICEF's goals to reduce world-population pressures—work toward meeting the obligations that we all share on this planet, our only home. W

Did You Know That . . .

One survey showed that 84 percent of respondents would opt for a lower, rather than higher, standard of living if it meant cleaner air, more pure drinking water, and a generally healthier environment.

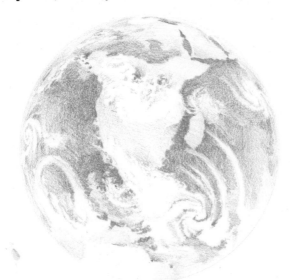

Glossary

A

Acid rain: Rain that contains relatively high concentrations of acid-forming air pollutants, such as sulfur and nitrogen oxides; acid rain may have a pH level as low as 2.8 (on a scale that ranges from 1 to 14) as compared to normal rain's pH of 6.

Air pollution: The contamination of the atmosphere by substances other than water.

Asbestos: A naturally occurring fibrous mineral that is widely used in insulating and fire-proofing materials; exposure to asbestos has been linked to lung cancer.

Asiatic cholera: An infection of the small intestine caused by the bacterium *Vibria cholerae* that results in severe, watery diarrhea, and in acute cases can lead to rapid dehydration and death if untreated; long confined to portions of South Asia, the disease has spread throughout the rest of the Third World and to the Gulf Coast of the United States since the 1950s.

C

Carbon cycle: The natural sequence through which carbon circulates in the biosphere; it begins with the conversion of atmospheric carbon dioxide to carbohydrates by plants; the carbon stored in plants is returned to the atmosphere in the form of carbon dioxide via one of several routes, including respiration (by animals that subsist on plants), the burning of fossil fuels (primarily coal and oil), or the eventual decomposition of plants, animals, and animal waste products.

Carbon monoxide (CO): A colorless, odorless gas formed as a by-product during the incomplete combustion of fossil fuels; it is also found in coal gas and in the exhaust of internal-combustion engines.

Carcinogenic: A term used to describe any substance or agent known to cause cancer (a carcinogen).

Chlorination: A widely used water purification process that involves the addition of a chlorine compound to disinfect drinking-water supplies.

Clinical ecology: A subfield of ecology concerned with the clinical effects of the environment on health.

Coliform bacteria: Any of several species of bacteria that inhabit the large intestine, and whose presence in water is an indicator of pollution from human waste.

D

DDT: The common abbreviation for the chemical name of a colorless, crystalline, organic pesticide (dichloro-diphenyl-trichloroethane), first used in 1939, that disorganizes the nervous systems of a variety of insects on contact; because of its toxic effects on other forms of wildlife, all nonessential uses of DDT have been banned in the United States and many other countries.

Desalinization: The removal of salt and other substances from water (usually seawater) to make it drinkable; also known as desalination.

Desertification: The spread of desert to previously fertile areas, a process involving the rapid loss of topsoil and depletion of plant life; desertification is usually the result of the combined impact of drought and overuse and mismanagement of the land by humans.

Dosage: The quantity of a given substance associated with a given measurable or observable effect.

Doubling time: The interval required for a given population to double in size.

E

Ecological niche: The functional role of a given species within an ecosystem.

Ecology: The biological study of the relationship between living things and their environments; also known as environmental science.

Ecosystem: A dynamic community that comprises all of the living creatures and their total environment within a specified area.

F

Fixation: The process by which atmospheric- or soil-based nitrogen and carbon compounds are converted into new forms usable by living organisms.

Formaldehyde: A colorless, pungent gas that is both suffocating and poisonous in high dosages; formaldehyde is a component of a variety of resins and plastics that are widely used as building materials.

Fission: A process in which the nucleus of an atom is bombarded with neutrons so that it splits; in the cases of uranium and plutonium atoms this results in the release of enormous quantities of energy.

Fusion: The process in which light atomic nuclei combine (fuse) to form a heavier material, as when deuterium (a hydrogen isotope) nuclei are fused to form helium; the fusion process releases enormous amounts of energy and is the means by which the energy produced in the interior of stars is generated; to date, fusion has occurred on Earth only in hydrogen-bomb explosions.

G

Geothermal energy: Energy from deep within the Earth's crust, usually in the form of heat; this energy can be tapped in a variety of ways, including wells that convert water to steam, which is then used to drive generators.

Germ theory of disease: The theory that many diseases are caused by microorganisms such as bacteria, fungi, and viruses ("germs") that invade the bodies of larger organisms; this theory was proposed in the mid-19th century by the French scientist Louis Pasteur (1822–1895) and further developed by the German bacteriologist Robert Koch (1843–1910).

Greenhouse effect: The heating effect on the Earth caused when long-wave (infrared) radiation emitted from the Earth's surface is absorbed by trace gases (notably carbon dioxide and methane) in the atmosphere and partially radiated back to the Earth's surface.

H

Hydrologic cycle: The natural sequence through which water circulates in the biosphere; surface water passes into the Earth's atmosphere in the form of water vapor (via the process of evaporation), falls from the atmosphere in the form of rain, snow, or other precipitation, and ultimately returns to the atmosphere through evaporation.

L

Law of limiting factors: The biological law that the size of any population is ultimately limited by one or more environmental factors.

Leachate: A solution that results from the dissolving of soluble substances by downward-percolating groundwater.

Leaching: The process by which soluble substances found in the soil and in landfills are dissolved and carried away by groundwater.

Lead: A heavy, comparatively soft metal that is easy to work and most commonly found in nature combined as a sulfide; lead is poisonous when absorbed by the body.

M

Mutagenic: A term used to describe any substance or agent known to cause or increase the rate of genetic mutation; a mutagen.

N

Nitrate(s): The name applied to any member of two groups of compounds derived from nitric acid, known as nitric acid esters and nitric acid salts; also refers to fertilizers containing potassium nitrate or sodium nitrate.

Nitrite: Any of a class of compounds derived from nitrous acid; one of the most common of these is sodium nitrite, which is widely used to preserve and enhance the appearance of cured meats; various nitrites are commonly used in the manufacture of drugs, dyes, explosives, and other chemicals.

Nitrogen cycle: The natural sequence through which nitrogen circulates in the biosphere; nitrogen compounds in the soil are taken in and stored by plants; when the plants are eaten by animals, these compounds are broken down into a variety of new compounds and a portion passed as waste; along with nitrogen in the atmosphere, the nitrogen passed into the soil in this fashion (or by the decay of plants or animals) is then converted by nitrogen-fixing bacteria into nitrogen compounds used by plants.

Nitrogen dioxide (NO_2): A reddish-brown, highly poisonous gas present in the exhaust of internal-combustion engines that is a major air pollutant in many urban areas.

O

Ocean dumping: The practice of hauling solid waste into the ocean and dumping it in one or more locations.

Open dump: A place where solid waste (refuse, garbage, trash, and the like) is taken and left uncovered; also known as a dump site.

Oxidize(d): To combine an element or a compound with oxygen, thus converting it into an oxide.

P

Particulate matter: Solid or liquid particles that are suspended in the Earth's atmosphere, especially pollutants.

PCB(s): The common abbreviation of the chemical name polychlorinated biphenyl, which applies to several mixtures of organic compounds produced by the reaction of chlorine with biphenyl; widely used as lubricants and heat-transfer fluids in electrical equipment, especially transformers, PCBs are toxic and resist decomposition.

Pesticide(s): Any chemical or substance used to destroy one or more species of pests (usually insects); while some pesticides are natural in origin, most are man-made.

Photochemical reaction(s): A chemical reaction caused by the effects of light on one or more chemicals; photochemical reactions play a significant role in the formation of smog in many urban areas.

Photosynthesis: The chemical process by which green plants convert water and carbon dioxide into food using energy from sunlight.

Population(s): All the individuals from a particular species living in a given area.

R

Radon: A naturally occurring, radioactive, gaseous element that is a product of radium decay; high radon levels that build up in enclosed areas are a potential health hazard.

Replacement rate: The number of births within a given population over a given period of time (birth rate) required to offset the normal number of deaths expected to occur within that same population during that same period (mortality rate).

S

Sanitary landfill: An area of land built up from deposits of solid waste in layers covered by soil.

Secondhand smoke: Tobacco smoke that is inhaled by nonsmokers.

Smog: A dense mixture of smoke and fumes combined with fog that is formed when air pollutants (particularly exhaust from automobiles) are trapped at ground level by a temperature inversion; smog is most common in heavily urbanized or industrial areas.

Solar energy: Energy derived directly from the sun's rays; also refers to the direct conversion of energy from the sun to electrical energy or heat via any one of a variety of means, including liquid heat storage and photovoltaic (solar) cells.

Sulfur dioxide (SO_2): A colorless gas with a choking odor that is a by-product of the combustion of substances such as fossil fuels that contain sulfur; it is chiefly used in the manufacture of chemicals such as sulfuric acid.

Surface water: Water found in oceans, ponds, lakes, streams, wetlands, and such, on the Earth's surface.

T

Teratogenic: A term used to describe any substance or agent known to cause birth defects (a teratogen).

Threshold(s): A point on a continuum at which additional changes in the value of one or more variables lead to rapid change in other variables.

Toxic substances: Substances that are known to produce harmful or poisonous effects upon exposure, usually through interference with one or more of the chemical reactions that take place in living tissues.

Toxicity: The relative strength of a toxic substance; substances whose toxicity is high require only a small dosage to produce harmful effects.

Typhoid fever: An infectious disease contracted by eating food or drinking water contaminated with the bacterium *Salmonella typhosa;* the first symptom is usually severe headache, which is followed by fever, diarrhea or constipation, loss of appetite, and may progress to delir-

ium; typhoid fever usually clears up within 4 weeks but can be fatal if left untreated.

W

Water pollution: The contamination of water by impurities, including decaying organic matter, chemicals, dissolved gases, and suspended solids.

Water power: Power derived from tapping the fall or rush of water in rivers or streams via turbines, waterwheels, or other devices; future potential sources of water power include devices to harness the power of ocean currents and waves.

Watershed: The region drained by a stream, lake, or other body of water.

Wind power: Power derived from the flow of natural air currents; the most common wind-power device is the windmill.

Z

Zero population growth (ZPG): The maintenance of a given population at a constant level so that there is no growth in its size; ZPG advocates favor limiting births by encouraging families to have no more than some specified number of children, usually 2.

Notes

CHAPTER 1

1. G. Easterbrook, "Cleaning Up," *Newsweek,* 24 July 1989, 26–35.
2. J. J. Hanlon and G. E. Pickett, *Public Health Administration and Practice,* 6th ed. (St. Louis: Mosby, 1974), 14.
3. L. Shattuck, *Report of the Sanitary Commission of Massachusetts* (Boston: Dutton & Wentworth, 1850).
4. R. Carson, *Silent Spring* (Boston: Houghton Mifflin, 1962).
5. L. R. Brown and S. L. Postel, "Thresholds of Change," *The Futurist,* September–October 1987, 9–14.
6. G. 0. Barney, *The Global 2000 Report to the President of the United States: Entering the 21st Century,* vol. 1 (Elmsford, NY: Pergamon Press, 1980), 3–5.
7. A. Toufexis, "Overpopulation: Too Many Mouths," *Time,* 2 January 1989, 48–50.
8. The Global Tomorrow Coalition, *The Global Ecology Handbook: What You Can Do About the Environmental Crisis,* W. H. Carson, ed. (Boston: Beacon Press, 1990), 3.

CHAPTER 2

1. G. Richards, "How to Get the Poor Some Help," *The Humanist,* March/April 1986, 19–22.
2. R. Clarke, "The World Population Boom," *World Press Review,* April 1986, 42.
3. Clarke, p. 42.
4. M. M. Kent, *Family Size Preferences: Evidence From the World Fertility Surveys* (Washington, DC: Population Reference Bureau, 1982), 26.
5. R. E. Hamil, "The Arrival of the 5-Billionth Human," *The Futurist,* July–August 1987, 37.
6. A. Toufexis, "Overpopulation: Too Many Mouths," *Time,* 2 January 1989, 48–50.
7. T. R. Malthus, "An Essay on the Principle of Population as It Affects the Future Improvement of Society," in *Population, Evolution, & Birth Control,* Garrett Hardin, ed. (San Francisco: W. H. Freeman, 1969), 4–16.
8. Richards, p. 19.
9. D. H. Meadows et al., *The Limits to Growth* (New York: Universe Books, 1972).

10. L. F. LaRouche, Jr., *There Are No Limits to Growth* (New York: Benjamin Franklin House, 1983).

11. W. Fornos, "The Moral Implications of Our Population Policy," *The Humanist*, January–February 1987, 30–32.

12. L. R. Brown and S. L. Postel, "Thresholds of Change," *The Futurist*, September–October 1987, 9–14.

13. Address by Werner Fosnos, Pres. (Delivered at the Population Institute, Eugene, Oregon, 16 April 1991).

14. R. W. Fox, A. Carroll, and M. L. Prueitt, "Population Images," *The Futurist*, March–April 1988, 31.

15. "Stress' Effect on Immune System," *USA Today*, June 1989, 4.

16. R. Clarke, "The World Population Boom," *World Press Review*, April 1986, 42.

17. Fornos, pp. 30–32.

18. W. Steger and J. Bowermaster, *Saving the Earth: A Citizen's Guide to Environmental Action* (New York: A. A. Knopf, 1990).

19. J. Naar, *Design for a Livable Planet: How You Can Help Clean Up the Environment* (New York: HarperCollins, 1990), 127.

20. A. Ehrlich and P. Erlich, "The Population Bomb Revisited," in *Life After '80: Environmental Choices We Can Live With*, K. Courrier, ed. (Andover, MA: Brick House Publishing Company, 1980), 70.

21. S. Coffel, *But Not a Drop to Drink: The Lifesaving Guide to Good Water* (New York: Rawson Associates, 1989).

22. The Global Tomorrow Coalition, *The Global Ecology Handbook: What You Can Do About the Environmental Crisis*, W. H. Carson, ed. (Boston: Beacon Press, 1990), 192.

23. M. Rogers, "Alaska, The Future Is Now," *Newsweek*, 18 September 1989, 63–64.

24. Rogers, p. 63.

25. W. W. Eaton, "Solar Energy," in *Perspective on Energy*, 2d ed., C. C. Ruedisili and M. W. Firebaugh, eds. (New York: Oxford University Press, 1978).

CHAPTER 3

1. T. Pawlick, *A Killing Rain: The Global Threat of Acid Precipitation* (San Francisco: Sierra Club Books, 1984), 1.

2. E. P. Eckholm, *Down to Earth: Environment and Human Needs* (New York: W. W. Norton, 1982), 93.

3. P. ReVelle and C. ReVelle, *The Environment: Issues and Choices for Society* (Boston: PWS Publishers, 1981), 373.

4. M. B. McElroy, "The Challenge of Global Change," *Bulletin of the American Academy of Arts and Sciences* 42 (1989): 25–38.

5. P. D. Jones and T. M. L. Wigley, "Global Warming Trends," *Scientific American,* August 1990, 84.

6. R. A. Houghton and G. M. Woodwell, "Global Climatic Change," *Scientific American,* April 1989, 36.

7. See, for example, Houghton and Woodwell, p. 36, and A. Leaf, "Potential Health Effects of Global Climatic and Environmental Changes," *New England Journal of Medicine* 321, no. 23 (7 December 1989): 1578.

8. Houghton and Woodwell, p. 39.

9. S. Begley, M. Hager, and L. Wilson, "Is It All Hot Air?" *Newsweek,* 20 November 1989, 64–66.

10. T. E. Graedel and P. J. Crutzen, "The Changing Atmosphere," *Scientific American,* September 1989, 62.

11. G. Easterbrook, "Cleaning Up," *Newsweek,* 24 July 1989, 33.

12. ReVelle and ReVelle, p. 385.

13. A. Nadakavukaren, *Man & Environment: A Health Perspective* 2d ed. (Prospect Heights, IL: Waveland Press, 1986), 163.

14. A. Bredin, "On Ill Health and Air Pollution," *The Good Health Magazine,* a special issue of *New York Times Magazine,* 7 October 1990, 18.

15. Bredin, p. 19.

16. B. Carey, "A Jog in the Smog," *Hippocrates,* May/June 1989, 96.

17. Pawlick, p. 4.

18. R. Reinhold, "Frustrated by Global Efforts, City Fights Ozone on Its Own," *New York Times,* 19 July 1989, A12.

19. Graedel and Crutzen, p. 63.

20. L. R. Brown, *State of the World, 1989: A Worldwatch Institute Report on Progress Toward a Sustainable Society* (New York: W. W. Norton, 1989), 243.

21. Leaf, p. 1580.

22. "In Search of the Healthy Home," *Special Reports,* May–July 1989, 12.

23. L. Lamb, "Environmental Illness: The New Plague," *Utne Reader,* September–October 1989, 14–15.

24. C. Lockhead, "Pollutants Reined in by Market Rules," *Insight,* 3 July 1989, 9–15.

25. A. Milne, *Our Drowning World: Population, Pollution and Future Weather* (Bridgeport, England: Prism Press, 1988).

26. Easterbrook, p. 33.

27. Easterbrook, p. 29.

28. Easterbrook, p. 28.

CHAPTER 4

1. N. Berliner, "The Year of the Spills," *Environmental Action,* September/October 1989, 12–15.
2. J. Cousteau, "The Commandments of the Sea," in *Life After '80: Environmental Choices We Can Live With,* K. Courrier, ed. (Andover, MA: Brick House Publishing Company, 1980), 3.
3. G. T. Miller, Jr., *Living in the Environment* 4th ed. (Belmont, CA: Wadsworth Publishing Company, 1985), 358.
4. W. H. MacLeish, "Water, Water Everywhere, How Many Drops to Drink?" *World Monitor,* December 1990, 54–58.
5. D. Zwick, "Our Inland Waters," in *Life after '80: Environmental Choices We Can Live With,* K. Courrier, ed. (Andover, MA: Brick House Publishing Company, 1980), 13.
6. P. ReVelle and C. ReVelle, *The Environment: Issues and Choices for Society* (Boston: PWS Publishers, 1981), 93.
7. A. Nadakavukaren, *Man & Environment: A Health Perspective* 2d ed. (Prospect Heights, IL: Waveland Press, 1986), 163.
8. J. MacDonald, "Home Water Purifiers," *Garbage* (March/April 1991), 33.
9. ReVelle and ReVelle, p. 140.
10. "Fit to Drink," *Consumer Reports,* January 1990, 27–32.
11. J. W. Maurits la Rivière, "Threats to the World's Water," *Scientific American,* September 1989, 89.
12. J. W. Maurits la Rivière, p. 84.
13. "EPA Says Pesticides, Nitrates Taint Hundreds of Communities' Drinking Water," *The Sun,* Baltimore, MD, 14 November 1990, 11A.
14. ReVelle and ReVelle, pp. 117, 122.
15. S. Coffel, *But Not a Drop to Drink! The Lifesaving Guide to Good Water* (New York: Rawson Associates, 1989).
16. Coffel.
17. ReVelle and ReVelle, pp. 119–122.
18. M. Klockenbrink, "Cleansing Waters," *American Health,* September 1989, 72.
19. "Fit to Drink," *Consumer Reports,* January 1990, 27–32.
20. Cousteau, pp. 5–9.

CHAPTER 5

1. *Our Earth, Ourselves: The Action-Oriented Guide to Help You Protect and Preserve Our Planet* (New York: Bantam Books, 1990), 168.

2. M. Beck et al., "Buried Alive," *Newsweek,* 27 November 1989, 67.

3. J. Langone, "A Stinking Mess," *Time,* 2 January 1989, 44.

4. M. Beck et al., p. 68.

5. Langone, p. 45.

6. M. Beck et al., p. 67.

7. J. Naar, *Design for a Livable Planet: How You Can Help Clean Up the Environment* (New York: HarperCollins, 1990), 15.

8. J. M. Moran, *Introduction to Environmental Science* 2d ed. (San Francisco: W. H. Freeman, 1986).

9. "Stop the Trashing of America," *USA Today,* June 1989, 3.

10. Langone, p. 45.

11. R. A. Frosch and N. E. Gallopoulos, "Strategies for Manufacturing," *Scientific American,* September 1989, 144.

12. B. Breen, "Burn It?" *Garbage,* March–April 1991, 45.

13. "What's An Executive to Do?" *Industry Week,* 4 September 1989, 89.

14. C. McAllister, "Save the Trees—and You May Save a Bundle," *Business Week,* 4 September 1989, 118.

15. "Cash from Trash," *Fortune,* 19 June 1989, 16.

16. C. Pollock-Shea, "Recycling Urban Wastes: Solving the Garbage Glut," *USA Today,* July 1988, 88.

17. "Burning Question," *The Economist,* 28 May 1988, 29–32.

18. Pollock-Shea, p. 89.

19. United States Congress, Office of Technology Assessment, "Facing America's Trash: What Next for Municipal Solid Waste," OTA-0-424 (Washington, DC: Government Printing Office, October 1989).

20. Beck et al., pp. 69–70.

21. Langone, p. 47.

CHAPTER 6

1. M. Oppenheimer and R. H. Boyle, *Dead Heat: The Race Against the Greenhouse Effect* (New York: Basic Books, 1990).

2. C. Spencer, "Help Wanted: An Activist's Guide to a Better Earth," *Omni,* September 1989, 109–124.

3. L. W. Foderaro, "Trying to Hold Down the Garbage Pile," *New York Times,* 30 November 1990: B1–B2.

4. Foderaro, pp. B1–B2.

5. C. Libov, "We're Concerned About Cancer," *New York Times,* 19 March 1989, 23.

6. K. R. Smith, "Air Pollution: Assessing Total Exposure in the United States," *Environment* 30, no. 8 (October 1988), 37.

7. The Global Tomorrow Coalition, *The Global Ecology Handbook: What You Can Do About the Environmental Crisis,* W. H. Carson, ed. (Boston: Beacon Press, 1990), 170.

8. J. Naar, *Design for a Livable Planet: How You Can Help Clean Up the Environment* (New York: HarperCollins, 1990), 218.

9. Oppenheimer and Boyle.

10. Oppenheimer and Boyle.

11. M. Shodell, "Risky Business," *Science 85,* October 1985, 47.

Resources

BOOKS

Brown, Lester R., and the Worldwatch Institute. *The State of the World 1991*. New York: W. W. Norton & Co., 1991.

Issued annually, this volume reviews the state of the world environment. The issues addressed include sustainable agriculture, hunger, waste disposal, water supply and safety, transportation, land degradation, ozone destruction, and other critical environmental issues.

Cohen, Bernard L. *The Nuclear Energy Option: An Alternative for the 90s*. New York: Plenum Press, 1990.

Cohen argues in favor of nuclear energy to supply the increasing demand for electricity. He presents information to show that the safety factor in nuclear technology has very much improved and that the benefits of nuclear power, such as toxic emissions reduction, far outweigh the minimal risks of radiation poisoning or reactor accidents.

Commoner, Barry. *Making Peace with the Planet*. New York: Pantheon Books, 1990.

In this book the author addresses the progress and the failures of our modern civilization to control the damage done by technological growth and the resultant pollution. Commoner draws heavily on technical information and provides discussion and analysis of environmental action and regulation. Also discussed are population, the solid waste crisis, automobile emissions controls, mercury poisoning, the greenhouse effect, and "acceptable risk" calculations.

Dadd, Debra Lynn. *The Nontoxic House: Protecting Yourself and Your Family From Everyday Toxics and Health Hazards*. Los Angeles: J. P. Tarcher, 1986.

The average house in the United States is filled with toxic chemicals—from cleansers to personal care items, from food and clothing to wall-to-wall carpeting. All these toxins, the author states, have been linked to headaches, depression, sterility, diseases of the nervous system, cancers, birth defects, and genetic abnormalities. The book works as a consumer's guide to selecting safe household products.

Environment '90: The Legislative Agenda. Washington, DC: Congressional Quarterly, 1990.

This book covers recent developments of the renewed environmental movement and provides discussions of statistics on such topics as clean air, energy, fuel economy, agriculture, timber, solid waste, nuclear arms, and recycling. The book addresses which environmental problems are considered to be the most serious by scientists and other professionals, and it reviews the U.S. government's stance on environmental protection.

Gough, Michael. *Dioxin, Agent Orange: The Facts*. New York: Plenum Press, 1986.

Gough presents a detailed and comprehensive argument showing the effects of dioxin on cancer in adults, birth defects in children, and deaths of Vietnam veterans. He also explains that dioxin is an unavoidable by-product in the manufacture of useful consumer products and is a result of the burning of wood, plastic, and garbage.

Gupte, Pranay. *The Crowded Earth: People and the Politics of Population*. New York: W. W. Norton, 1984.

The author interviewed leaders and common people on 5 continents to determine how the lives of people are shaped by population pressures and the related issues of health care, aging, migration, and urbanization. Although present population growth has slowed, Gupte warns that unless we understand the problem of population growth, a new population explosion will occur.

Jacobson, Michael. *Safe Food: Eating Wisely in a Risky World*. San Francisco: Living Planet Press, 1991.

This work, by the current executive director of the Center for Science in the Public Interest, is a carefully documented examination of the risks related to what we eat. An overview of the major food safety issues of the past 20 years is coupled with an analysis of which risks to be concerned about and which to ignore. The book also includes practical advice about the steps ordinary consumers can take to protect themselves against food-related risks. This is an extremely useful and timely work which encourages readers to feel they can and do have some control over their environment.

Roan, Sharon L. *Ozone Crisis: The 15-Year Evolution of a Sudden Global Emergency.* New York: John Wiley & Sons, 1989.

Science writer Roan chronicles the experiences of two scientists who first made the discovery that the widespread release of chlorofluorocarbons (CFCs) into the air was causing Earth's protective ozone layer to disintegrate. She explores the resistance of government, world leaders, and manufacturers of CFCs to accept this information, and provides insights into what future action must be taken to preserve the layer of ozone that protects the Earth from the sun's harmful ultraviolet radiation.

Schneider, Stephen H. *Global Warming: Are We Entering the Greenhouse Century?* San Francisco: Sierra Club Books, 1989.

This book examines the causes of worldwide climatic change that some scientists predict will raise the Earth's average temperature by 10° Fahrenheit in less than a century. A rise in sea level, extensively altered weather patterns, and crop failures are just some of the repercussions of such a dramatic environmental change. Schneider outlines definitive ways in which individuals, governments, and businesses can cooperate to slow the damage of global technological development and population growth.

Stellman, Jeanne, and Mary Sue Henifin. *Office Work Can Be Dangerous to Your Health.* New York: Pantheon, 1983.

Although dated, this book contains valuable safety information on office air pollution from photocopy machines and other common office machinery. The hidden effects of faulty office design are also addressed, such as inadequate ventilation, temperature control, and lighting. Information is provided on topics from allergies and back pain to factors that can cause sprained ankles and even broken bones. The authors present detailed discussions and solutions.

Sullivan, Julie, ed. *The American Environment.* New York: H. W. Wilson, 1984.

This book provides a detailed review of the Reagan administration's drastic change in the Environmental Protection Agency's policy from strict to less stringent controls. The Reagan policy, the author states, was to reduce the

level of governmental control by giving more power to industry and the private sector in regulating pollution. This pro-economy stance resulted in less healthful air and water and greater health risks for our society. The book provides a comprehensive analysis of how government, industry, and environmental groups can cooperate to generate economic growth with the least negative impact on our health and on the environment.

Tollison, Robert D., ed. *Clearing the Air: Perspectives on Environmental Tobacco Smoke.* Lexington, MA: D. C. Heath, 1988.

Presented here is the hard scientific evidence that lets the reader draw his or her own conclusions about the health effects of environmental tobacco smoke. The editor has compiled a full range of evidence and points of view to provide a well-balanced perspective on the issues of environmental tobacco smoke. Perspectives include those of health professionals, an economist, a sociologist, a labor union official, and a corporate president. Chapters include discussion of public-health programs, cigarettes and property rights, and perspectives from the workplace, the press, and politics.

PERIODICALS

Baseline is published monthly for free and provides nontechnical information about current environmental policies and programs in the State of Washington. Each issue also explores various emerging and existing environmental issues and trends. Write to the Department of Ecology, Public Affairs Office, Olympia, WA 98504-8711.

Environ is published quarterly and provides resource information for purchasing products that are environmentally sound, lists companies that operate with attention to a healthy environment, and updates readers on the latest research in environmental health. For a one-year subscription, which is $15, write *Environ*, P.O. Box 2204, Fort Collins, CO 80522, or call (303) 224-0083.

Environment is published monthly by Heldref Publications, a division of the nonprofit Helen Dwight Reid Foundation. Feature articles cover all issues regarding the world environment. Also provided is information on efficient energy use, recycling, air quality in cities, and other topics of interest to individuals on a local scale. A one-year subscription costs $24. To subscribe, write *Envi-*

ronment, 4000 Albemarle Street, NW, Washington, DC 20016, or call toll free (800) 365-9753.

Environmental Action is published bimonthly and covers information on acid rain, air pollution from industry and automobiles, water and soil contamination, and the actions of government, private industry, and private organizations to deal effectively with assaults on the environment. A one-year subscription costs $25. Write Environmental Action, Inc., 1525 New Hampshire Avenue, NW, Washington, DC 20036, or call (202) 745-4875.

Environmental Review is published quarterly and seeks to understand the human experience in relation to the environment. Emphasis is on the perspectives of history and the liberal arts and sciences. A subscription is $24 a year for individuals, $12 for students and retirees. Write American Society for Environmental History, c/o Center for Technology Studies, New Jersey Institute of Technology, Newark, NJ 07102, or call (201) 596-3270.

Garbage: The Practical Journal for the Environment covers such environmental issues as recycling, composting, garbage disposal, and energy conservation, and provides practical information for the interested layperson. A one-year subscription is $21. Write *Garbage,* Subscription Department, P.O. Box 56520, Boulder, CO 80321-6520.

Human Ecologist is published quarterly and provides information on human response to the environment. It explains how chemicals found in the air, water, food, drugs, pesticides, and habitat can result in environmental illness. A one-year subscription is $20. Write Human Ecology Action League, Box 66637, Chicago, IL 60666, or call (312) 665-6575.

Priorities: For Long Life & Good Health is published quarterly by the American Council on Science and Health, Inc. (ACSH), a nonprofit consumer education association promoting scientifically balanced evaluations of nutrition, chemicals, life-style factors, the environment, and human health. General individual membership in ACSH, which includes a subscription to *Priorities,* costs $25 a year. Write to the Subscription Department, *Priorities,* 1995 Broadway, 16th Floor, New York, NY 10023-5860.

World Monitor is published monthly by The Christian Science Publishing Society and often presents both feature and brief articles on topics related to health and the condition of the environment. A yearly subscription is $29.94. Write The Christian Science Publishing Society, One Norway Street, Boston, MA 02115, or call (800) 888-6261.

World • Watch is published 6 times a year by the Worldwatch Institute. The magazine covers environmental health issues from saving wetlands and cleaning up litter to nuclear energy issues and the growth of the hole in the Earth's ozone layer. A one-year subscription is $15. Write Worldwatch Institute, 1776 Massachusetts Avenue, NW, Washington, DC 20036.

HOTLINES

Environmental Protection Agency (EPA) Hotline, (800) 425-4791. Callers can obtain answers or referrals regarding questions about contaminants in air, water, and soil.

National Health Information Center House, Department of Health and Human Services, (800) 336-4797; in Maryland, call (301) 656-4167. This information and referral center is operated by the Office of Disease Prevention and Health Promotion; its trained personnel will direct you to the organization or governmental agency that can assist you with your questions about air, water, waste disposal, and other environmental-health issues. Its hours are 9:00 A.M. to 5:00 P.M., Eastern Standard Time, Monday through Friday.

GOVERNMENT, CONSUMER, AND ADVOCACY GROUPS

American Council on Science and Health (ACSH), 1995 Broadway, 16th Floor, New York, NY 10023, (212) 362-7044

This group's purpose is to provide consumers with information on food, chemicals, the environment, and human health. Council personnel participate in government regulatory proceedings, public debates, and other forums and provide articles regularly for professional and scientific journals and popular media. The council holds national press conferences; produces a syndicated series of health updates for radio; has a 24-hour, computerized information telephone line providing commentary, press releases, and questions and answers on health topics; and publishes brochures and research reports on numerous health topics, including risks and benefits regarding public health and environmental issues.

American Lung Association (ALA), 1740 Broadway, New York, NY 10019, (212) 315-8700

Membership includes a federation of state and local associations of physicians, nurses, and laypeople interested in the prevention and control of lung disease. ALA works with other organizations in research as well as planning and conducting programs in community services and public, professional, and hospital-patient education. It makes policy recommendations regarding medical care of respiratory diseases, occupational health, hazards of smoking, and air conservation; it produces several free brochures on indoor air pollution.

Asbestos Victims of America (AVA), P.O. Box 559, Capitola, CA 95010, (408) 476-3646

Members include individuals suffering from asbestos-related diseases, families and friends of asbestos victims, and those concerned about the hazards of asbestos. The group has been endorsed by union members. The goals of the AVA are to assist asbestos victims and their families in solving related medical, emotional, and financial problems, and to prevent further asbestos-related diseases through increased awareness. ALA provides referrals to doctors and attorneys and publishes newsletters, fact sheets, and pamphlets on this issue.

Cause For Concern (CC), R.D. 1, Box 570, Stewartsville, NJ 08886, (201) 479-4110

This environmental-education organization of parents and concerned citizens encourages consumers to purchase nontoxic household products as alternatives to toxic equivalents. CC works with other environmental organizations and publishes newsletters and fact sheets.

Center For Health Action (CHA), P.O. Box 270, Forest Park Station, Springfield, MA 01108, (413) 782-2115

Membership comprises individuals opposed to fluoridation of U.S. drinking water; seeks to implement control programs for the addition of fluoride to water; and acts as a clearinghouse, collecting and disseminating information on the effects of low-level fluoride on our health.

Citizens Against Tobacco Smoke (CATS), P.O. Box 36236, Cincinnati, OH 45236, (513) 984-8834

Membership includes health and environmental organizations and individuals concerned with indoor air pollution caused by tobacco smoke. The organization has set a national

agenda for a tobacco-free society by the year 2000 and supports a smoking ban in enclosed public places, restaurants, and workplaces. CATS sponsors the Smoke-Free Skies campaign, which supports a total ban on smoking on airline flights and in airports and disseminates information on the effects of second-hand smoke and on how to lobby for clean indoor air laws. It compiles statistics and publishes a quarterly newsletter for members.

Citizen's Clearinghouse for Hazardous Wastes (CCHW), P.O. Box 926, Arlington, VA 22216, (703) 276-7070

Membership includes individuals who live near or are concerned with hazardous waste dumps and the health effects on adults and children from contact with toxic chemicals and other hazardous wastes. CCHW provides information on and guidance in dealing with this environmental problem; representatives visit sites to determine the severity of the situation and pressure lawmakers to take action. It also conducts research on chemicals to determine dangerous levels of exposure, maintains a 2,000-volume library on waste-management technology, and publishes *Action Bulletin* and *Everyone's Backyard* quarterly and over 50 additional titles yearly.

Environmental Action (EA), 1525 New Hampshire Avenue, NW, Washington, DC 20036, (202) 745-4870

This group is a national political lobby working to control and reduce toxic substances, plutonium production, ozone-layer destruction, global warming, solid waste, and acid rain production and to improve drinking water, air quality, and to promote recycling. EA publishes *Environmental Action* bimonthly.

Environmental Defense Fund (EDF), 257 Park Avenue South, New York, NY 10010, (212) 5050-2100

Membership includes lawyers, scientists, and economists dedicated to the protection and improvement of environmental quality and public health. Their goal is to encourage responsible oversight and public policy in the administration of toxic chemical regulations, radiation control, and standards for air quality, energy conservation, water resources, and agriculture; their concerns focus on ozone depletion, global warming, protection of wildlife, and the international environment. EDF initiates legal action and litigation in environment-related matters and conducts public-service and education campaigns.

Environmental Health Watch (EHW), 4115 Bridge Avenue, Cleveland, Ohio, 44113 (216) 961-4646

The efforts of this group include the Healthy House Project, which educates and assists families concerned about the health effects of formaldehyde in carpets, asbestos in fireproofing materials and linoleum floors, lead in paint, pesticides, and other possibly polluting materials and products in the home.

Group Against Smokers' Pollution (GASP), P.O. Box 632, College Park, MD 20740, (301) 577-6427

Founded by nonsmokers whose health has been adversely affected by tobacco smoke, GASP's goal is to promote the rights of nonsmokers, to educate the public about the problems of secondhand smoke, and to regulate smoking in public places. It produces an educational slide series; distributes educational literature, buttons, posters, and bumper stickers; and publishes a handbook called *The Nonsmokers' Liberation Guide*.

Housing Resource Center (HRC), 1820 West 48th Street, Cleveland, OH 44102, (216) 281-4663

This nonprofit organization provides consumers with practical information on home maintenance and repair and ways to promote a healthy home environment. HRC publishes *Your Home* newsletter quarterly and answers telephone queries about health improvement projects in the home.

Human Ecology Action League (HEAL), P.O. Box 66637, Chicago, IL 60666, (312) 665-6575

Members comprise individuals and organizations interested in the study of human ecology and human illness as affected by synthetic and natural substances in the environment. HEAL collects and disseminates information and works to eliminate or reduce conditions in the environment that are hazardous to human health. It publishes *Human Ecologist* quarterly, in addition to other publications, brochures, and newsletters.

Industrial Health Foundation (IHF), 34 Penn Circle, W., Pittsburgh, PA 15206, (412) 363-6600

IHF operates a laboratory that studies the prevention of industrial diseases and the improvement of working conditions. It offers continuing education programs and provides extensive information on disease-control procedures, health hazards, and toxicity; maintains a 1,300-volume library and bibliographical archives; publishes *Industrial Hygiene Digest* monthly and technical papers for engineers and scientists in the field of industrial health.

National Association of Nonsmokers (NANS), 8701 Georgia Avenue, Suite 200, Silver Spring, MD 20910-3714, (202) NO-SMOKE

This new nonprofit association was founded to represent the nonsmoker. The purpose of NANS is to support and promote responsible nonsmoking legislation, to educate the public about the relationship of smoking to health, and to assist members regarding their rights as nonsmokers. Interested individuals can become members for an annual fee of $10. Membership dues and contributions provide funds for promoting nonsmoking education and lobbying for nonsmokers' rights. The group's primary adviser is Cyril F. Brickfield, former president of the American Association of Retired Persons.

National Environmental Health (NEHA), 720 South Colorado Boulevard, Suite 970, South Tower, Denver, CO 80222, (303) 756-9090

This is a society of professionals from public and governmental health agencies, industry, colleges, and universities who share a concern for environmental health education. NEHA promotes educational efforts via colleges and universities and conducts continuing education programs. It publishes numerous newsletters, brochures, manuals, and reports.

National Water Center (NWC), P.O. 264, Eureka Springs, AR 72632, (501) 253-9755

Membership includes individuals interested in the maintenance and conservation of water resources. NWC seeks to increase public awareness of the need to protect sources of unpolluted water. It disseminates information on water-conservation techniques; offers consulting services to individuals and communities for methods of detoxifying wastes and protecting water resources; maintains a 300-volume library; and publishes *Water Center News* quarterly, plus books on sewage disposal and water pollution. The center also produces audiocassette tapes. Its videocassette tapes include *Heal the Waters, Wastewater Blues,* and *We All Live Down-Stream.*

Safe Water Coalition (SWC), 150 Woodland Avenue, San Anselmo, CA 94960, (415) 453-0158

Members include organizations, laypersons, and professionals who seek to inform the public on the toxic effects of fluoride in public water systems and in dental hygiene products. SWC collects information on fluoride research and statistics and publishes *National Fluoridation News* quarterly.

Tobacco Products Liability Project (TPLP), 400 Huntington Avenue, Northeastern University School of Law, Boston, MA 02115, (617) 437-2026

This is an autonomous project of the Clean Indoor Air Educational Foundation that is comprised of doctors, lawyers, public-health officials, and academics. It encourages liability suits against the tobacco industry in order to compensate victims of tobacco-related diseases and injuries such as cancers and burns, discourage tobacco smoking, and publicize its effects on health. This group also acts as an information clearinghouse, and publishes *Tobacco on Trial* 10 times a year, which covers product-liability cases against tobacco companies.

White Lung Association (WLA), 1114 Cathedral, Baltimore, MD 21201, (301) 727-6029.

Membership includes 10,000 individuals who organize self-help support groups for those suffering from exposure to asbestos. WLA serves as a clearinghouse, providing information on legal and medical assistance to asbestos victims and interested persons. It also conducts investigations and surveys of suspected contamination, and monitors the removal of asbestos in workplaces. It publishes *Asbestos Watch* semiannually.

Women's Occupational Health Resource Center (WOHRC), 117 Saint John's Place, Brooklyn, NY 11217, (718) 230-8822

The center functions as a clearinghouse for women's occupational health and safety issues. Their goal is to increase awareness of the health and safety hazards women face in the workplace, and to raise managerial awareness of the need for improved workplace conditions and for safer equipment design. WOHRC advises manufacturers on design standards of safety equipment; offers technical assistance in setting up programs designed to develop occupational health awareness; and publishes a quarterly newsletter, *WOHRC News,* in addition to fact sheets and bibliographies.

Index

Boldface page numbers refer to the pages in which the terms are defined.

A

abortion, 25
acid rain: **46**–48; caused by incineration, 97
advocacy, environmental, 111–112, 119–123
aerosol cans, 54, 55, 118
Africa: food and population in, 28–29; population growth of, 19–20, 24
age distribution, of population 21, 23
agriculture: slash-and-burn, 30–31; waste, 90
air pollution: **38**–63; and health, 51, 54–55; history of, 40, 42
Alaska, and oil, 35
alternative-fuel vehicles, in Los Angeles, 111
aluminum, 72, 90
American Lung Association of California, 51
Amicus Journal, 60
Antarctica, "hole" in the ozone layer over, 55
ANWR, *see* Arctic National Wildlife Refuge
apples, and expectations, 112–113
Arctic National Wildlife Refuge (ANWR), 35
asbestos, 49, **57**
ash disposal, from incineration, 98
Asiatic cholera, **74**
athletes, and air pollution, 51
atmosphere, and water, 7
attitudes, toward the environment, 111–112, 119–123
automobile: air conditioner, 54; emissions, 42, 50, 63, 111; interior pollution, 43

B

bacteria: coliform, 74–75; and nitrogen cycle, 9–10
Bangladesh, special programs for women in, 25
benzene, 43
biomass fuel, 35–36
biotic reorganization, 114–115
birth control efforts, in the Third World, 22–23, 24–25, 26
birth rates, 22

"bound water," 65
"business-as-usual pollution," 119

C

cadmium, 70
California: and air pollution, 51; *see also,* Los Angeles
cancer: lung, and air pollution, 51; skin, and ultraviolet radiation, 54–55
car, *see* automobile
carbohydrates, 8
carbon: 4; filter, 81, 82
carbon cycle, 8
carbon dioxide: 33, 44–46, 115; in the Earth's atmosphere, 11
carbon filter, 81, 82
carbon monoxide (CO), **42**–44
carcinogenic, **102**
Carson, Rachel, 6
Carter, U.S. president Jimmy, 12, 106
CFCs, *see* chlorofluorocarbons
charcoal filters, 82, 83
chemical(s): hazardous household, 116–119; and indoor pollution, 58–59; sensitivities, 59; waste, 87–88; in water, 69
children, and air pollution, 51
China, "one-family, one-child" policy in, 26
chlorination, **77**
chlorine, in the atmosphere, 52
chlorofluorocarbons (CFCs), 39, 50–56
cities: and air pollution, 43; and population, 29; and smog, 49–50
clean air, 38
Clean Air Act of 1970 and 1977, 62
Clean Water Act, 85
clinical ecology, **56**
"Club of Rome Report," *see The Limits to Growth*
coal, 34, 47–48
Coats, U.S. Sen. Dan, 92
coffee filters, unbleached paper, 112
coliform bacteria, **74**–75
Common Future, Our, 14
"Commons, The Tragedy of the," 11, 12
composting, in France, 99

conservation, 115
consumers: attitudes of, 111–112; recycling, 98; solutions for, 53–54, 115, 119–123
contraception, 24–25
copper, 72
corrosive products, 116–119
Cousteau, Jacques, 85
"curbside separation program," 96

D

DDT (dichloro-diphenyl-trichloro-ethane), **73**–74
demographics, 16, 18, 22
desalinization, **67**
desertification, **14**, 30
detoxing, 115
developed countries, 20–21
dichloro-diphenyl-trichloro-ethane, *see* DDT
dioxins, 97–98, 112
disease, caused by contaminated water, 74
disposal: ash, 98; of household hazardous chemicals, 118–119; toxic waste, 103
distillers, 81–82, 83
distribution: worldwide, of water, 65–66
dosage, **39**–40
doubling time, **21**
drinking water: 64–67; 75–85; EPA's, hotline, 81
drought, 66–67
dump: Fresh Kills, 92, 95; open, 90; town, 90; *see also,* landfills

E

Earth, and its relationship to life, 3
ecological niche, **6**
ecology: **6**; clinical, 56
ecosystem, **6**
Ehrlich, Anne and Paul, 32
elderly, worldwide, population, 13
electromagnetic radiation, 58
emissions: industrial, 32; automobile, 42, 50, 63, 111
energy: efficiency and indoor pollution, 56, 58–59; nonrenewable, sources, 34; and population, 34; renewable, sources, 35–37; transfer of, and materials, 10–11; from waste,

95–98; *see also,* individual forms

environmental illness, 60

Environmental Protection Agency (EPA): 55, 62–63, 80; drinking-water hotline, 81; and PCBs, 103

environmental resistance, 17

EPA, *see* Environmental Protection Agency

equilibrium, of population and environment, 17

Essay on the Principle of Population as It Affects the Future Improvement of Society, An, 27

exhaust, automobile, 42, 50, 63, 111

exposure, to a toxic substance, 39–40

extinction of species, 17

Exxon *Valdez,* 64

F

family planning, in the Third World, 22–23, 24–25, 26

FAO, *see* Food and Agricultural Organization fertilizers, as a water pollutant, 73–74

filter, water: 80, 82; carbon, 82

fission, 36–**37**

fixation, **8**, 9

food: and population density, 27–29, 30; and population growth, 24; production of, 13

Food and Agricultural Organization (FAO), of the United Nations, 29–30

forecasting population growth, 18

formaldehyde, **57**–60

fossil fuels, 34, 42

France, recycling in, 99

fraud, home water treatment, 78, 80–81

Fresh Kills Dump, 92, 95

fruit, and pesticides, 113

fuels, 35–36

fusion, **37**

G

garbage: 86–97, 100, 104–106; in Japan, 100; out- of-state, 91–93

gas, *see* natural gas

geothermal energy, **36**

germ theory of disease, **5**

"glasphalt," 99–100

glass recycling, 99–100

global warming: 62, 108–109; and the greenhouse effect, 44–46; and trees, 33

Global 2000 Report to the President of the United States: Entering the 21st Century, The, 12

Godish, Thad, 58

Good, Clint, 59

government, actions of, to manage resources, 32

Grace, W. R., plant, and water pollution, 76

greenhouse effect: **44**–46, 55; and weather, 46

H

halons: 53; fire extinguisher, 54

Hardin, Garrett, 11, 12, 28

hazardous waste: 101–103, 106–107; disposal of household, 118–119

health risks from: aluminum, 72; asbestos, 49, 57; cadmium, 70; copper, 72; formaldehyde, 58; incineration ash, 97; lead, 49; mercury, 70; outdoor air pollutants, 42–44; overpopulation, 37; ozone, 50; secondhand smoke, 60; sulfur dioxide, 48; toxic waste, 102

"Healthful Houses," 59

hearing, and noise pollution, 41

Hippocrates, 74

history: of air pollution, 40, 42; of incineration, 96–97; of indoor pollution, 56–57; of lead as a pollutant, 69–70; of public health movement, 4–6; of purifying water, 76–77

"hole," in the ozone layer, 55

homes, radon in, 59

home water treatment: 80–83; fraud in, 78, 80–81

Hooker Chemical and Plastics Corporation, 103, 106

Houghton, Richard, 45–46

household waste, 89–90

humankind: and air pollution, 38, 46; and the ecosystem, 16; and the environment, 1–2, 6, 12; impact on Earth, 3–4, 6, 14, 15; and indoor environment, 56; and the transfer of energy and materials, 10–11; and water, 32–34, 68

hydrochloric acid, 97–98

hydrogen chloride, 97–98

hydrologic cycle, 7, **64**

I

ignitable products, 116–119

incineration: 95–98; disadvantages, of, 97

Indiana, and garbage, 92

individual actions, 53–54, 84–85, 104–106, 111–112, 119–120

indoor pollution, history of, 56–57

industry: actions of, to manage resources, 32; emissions by, 32; energy needs of, 34; recycling by, 98

inorganic pollutants, 69–72; *see also,* individual forms

insulation, 54

International Human Suffering Index, 13–14

interstate movement of municipal solid waste, 91–93

ion-exchange softeners, 83

J

Japan, recycling in, 99

Jones, Philip, 45

juice boxes, 112

K

Kentucky, Benton, sewage treatment plant, 79

L

landfills: 87–88; at Love Canal, 103, 106–107; sanitary, 94; secure, 103

LaRouche, Lyndon, 28

law of limiting factors, **6**

leachate, **94**

leaching, **102**

lead, 49, **60**, 69–70, 81, 82

less developed countries, 19–20, 21, 22

life, and its relationship to the Earth, 3

limiting factors, law of, 6

Limits to Growth, The, 28

logging, 32

London, smog in, 42, 47–48

Los Angeles: benzene in, 43; smog in, 49, 51, 111; and trees, 115, 119

Love Canal, 103, 106–107

lung(s): cancer, 51; and smog, 50, 51; *see also,* cancer

M

Mali, 28
Malthus, Thomas Robert, 27–28
manufacturers, and recycling, 112
mass burn, 97
Massachusetts, water pollution
    in, 76–77, 80
Meade, Gladys, 51
melanoma, 54; *see also,* cancer
mercury, 70
Mexico City, population of, 24, 29
mining waste, 90
minerals, 32
Missouri, and garbage, 91, 93
Mobro, 88
Montreal Protocol, 56
Moynihan, U.S. Sen. Daniel
    Patrick, 32
mutagenic, **102**

N

National Safety Council, on
    hazardous household chemicals,
    118
National Solid Wastes
    Management Association
    (NSWMA), 91, 92
natural gas, 35
nature, and air pollution, 38
New Jersey: and chlorination, 77;
    and garbage, 91–92
New York: garbage in, City,
    86–88, 92; Love Canal, 103,
    106–107
New York City, and garbage,
    86–88, 92
NIMBY (Not In My Back Yard),
    88
nitrate(s), **9**–10, **74**, 81
nitrite, **10**
nitrogen, 9
nitrogen cycle, 9
nitrogen dioxide (NO2), **60**
nitrogen oxides, 50
noise pollution, 41
nonrenewable energy sources,
    34–35
Norplant, 25
nuclear energy, 36–37

O

ocean dumping, **90**, 94
oil, 34–35, 72
oil spills, 64
"one-family, one-child" policy in
    China, 26
open dump, **90**

organic pollutants: 72–74, 103;
    volatile, 81
out-of-state garbage, 91–93
outdoor air pollution, *see* air
    pollution
oxidize(d), **9**
ozone: 50–56; and health, 50,
    54–55
ozone layer, 50–56

P

packaging, 89–90, 97, 112
paint, with lead, 60
paper: vs. plastic, 104; recycling,
    98, 99, 100; as waste, 101
particulate matter, **48**–49
PCBs (polychlorinated biphenyls),
    69, 72–73, 103
Pelicano, 88
pesticides, **69**, 73–74, 81, 102, 113
Phalen, Robert, 51
photochemical reaction(s), **49**–50
photosynthesis, **9**
plants: and the carbon cycle, 8;
    and the nitrogen cycle, 10
plastic vs. paper, 104
pollutants: air, 39; inorganic,
    69–72; organic, 72–74; water,
    69
pollution: air, 38–63, 115; noise,
    41; water, 67–75, 76
polychlorinated biphenyls, *see*
    PCBs
polystyrene, 54
polyvinyl chlorides, *see* PVCs
population(s): **6**; age distribution
    of, 21, 23; control in the Third
    World, 22–23, 24–26; and
    energy, 34; and environment,
    17; and food, 27–29, 30;
    forecasting growth, 18; growth,
    12, 14; and health, 37; and
    water, 33–34
Population Crisis Committee, 13
"population pyramid," 21
"precursors," 38
precycling, 112
public health movement, history
    of, 4–6
PVCs, 97–98, 104

R

radon: 59, **60**; in water, 72, 81
Randolph, Pheron, 58–59
reactive products, 116–119
Reagan administration,
    antiabortion policy of, and the
    Third world, 25

recycling: 96–97, 98–101,
    104–106, 122; in France, 99;
    glass, 99–100; in Japan, 99,
    100; paper, 98, 99, 100; in the
    United States, 99, 100
reduction, 96–97
reforestation, 32
refrigerators, 54
religion, and population-control
    efforts, 23, 25
Renew America, 119–120
renewable energy sources, 35–37
replacement rate, 18–19
resource recovery plants, 94–98
resources: management of, 31–37;
    of the world and population,
    27–29
reverse-osmosis units, 82, 83
RU 486, 25
rural areas: and nitrates, 74; and
    sewage treatment, 77, 79

S

safe drinking water, 75–85
Safe Drinking Water Act, 80, 84
sand filters, 76–77
sanitary landfill, **94**
Sanitation Utilization Company,
    96
scrubbers, 97
secondhand smoke, **60**
secure landfills, 103
sewage-treatment plant: 77; in
    Benton, Kentucky, 79
shortages, of water, 66–67
"sick building syndrome," 56
"sick house syndrome," 58
skin cancer, and ultraviolet
    radiation, 54–55; *see also,*
    cancer
slash-and-burn agriculture, 30–31
smog: **47**–48; and health, 51,
    54–55; in London, 42;
    photochemical, in Los Angeles,
    49–50, 51
smoke: secondhand, 60; tobacco,
    42
solar energy: **36;** and the
    greenhouse effect, 44
solid waste: 86–107; interstate
    movement of municipal, 91–93;
    toxic, 101–103, 106–107
solutions: for individuals, 84–85,
    111–112, 115, 119–123; for
    nations, 26
sound, as noise pollution, 41
Star Recycling, 92–93
sterilization, 25

sulfur dioxide (SO$_2$), **46**–48
sulfur trioxide (SO$_3$), 48
surface water, **7**

T

Tennessee Valley Authority
    (TVA), and sewage treatment,
    77, 79
teratogenic, **102**
testing water, 80–82
TFR, *see* total fertility rate
There Are No Limits to Growth,
    28
Third World: population control
    in, 22–23, 24–25, 26;
    population growth in, 18,
    19–20
THMs, *see* trihalomethanes
Thompson, Warren, 16
threshold(s), **6**
total fertility rate (TFR), 18–20
town dump, 90
towns, small, and sewage
    treatment, 77, 79
toxic substances, **38**, 116–119
toxic waste: 87–88, 101–103,
    106–107; sites, 107
toxicity, **39**–40, 102
transfer rates, of energy and
    materials, 10–11
transfer stations, 92–93
trash, 86–88
trash-to-energy plants, 95–98
treatment, home water: 80–83;
    devices for, 82–83; fraud in, 78,
    80–81

trees, and carbon dioxide, 33,
    115, 119
trihalomethanes (THMs), 81, 82
trucking out-of-state garbage,
    91–93
TVA, *see* Tennessee Valley
    Authority
typhoid fever, **74**

U

ultraviolet (UV) rays, 53, 54
United Nations: and the
    environment, 14; Food and
    Agricultural Organization
    (FAO), 29–30; population
    forecast, 12
United States, recycling in, 99
urban centers: and air pollution,
    43; and population, 29; and
    smog, 49–50

V

VOCs, *see* volatile organic
    compounds
Vohra, Shri B. B., 13, 24
volatile organic compounds
    (VOCs), 81

W

Waring, Col. George E., Jr., 96
waste: -to-energy facility, 95–98;
    solid, 86–107; toxic, 87–88,
    101–103, 106–107
"waste chain," 103

Waste Information Network, 93
waste-to-energy facility, 95–98
wastewater treatment, 77, 79
water: in the atmosphere, 7;
    conservation, 115; drinking,
    64–67, 75–85; fraud in home,
    treatment, 78, 80–81, 82–83;
    necessity of, to humans, 32–34;
    pollution, 67–75; quality,
    68–69; testing, 80–82;
    worldwide distribution of,
    65–66
water filter, 80, 82–83
water pollution: **67**–75, 76
water power, **36**
watershed, **7**
weather, and the greenhouse
    effect, 46
wetlands, and sewage treatment,
    79
Wigley, Tom, 45
Wilcox, Bruce, 25
wind power, **36**
women, social status of, and
    family planning, 25
Woodwell, George, 45–46
World Commission on
    Environment and Development,
    14

Z

zero population growth (ZPG), **18**
ZPG, *see* zero population growth

Page 3 Copyright © October 31, 1988, *U.S. News & World Report.* Page 11 Reprinted from *Science* magazine, Vol. 162, 1968, with permission from Garrett Hardin. Page 14 From *The Global Ecology Handbook.* Copyright © 1990 by the Global Tomorrow Coalition, used by permission of Beacon Press, Boston. Page 22 Table 2.1 Reprinted with permission from Waveland Press, Inc. Page 24 Copyright © 1988 Time Warner Inc. Reprinted by permission. Page 33 From *Design for a Livable Planet: How You Can Help Clean Up the Environment,* by J. Naar. Copyright © 1990 by J. Naar. Reprinted by permission of HarperCollins Publishers. Page 43 By Katherine Griffin. Reprinted from *In Health,* copyright © 1989. Page 51 Reprinted from *American Health,* copyright © 1989 by J.E. Basu. Page 53 Reprinted with permission of *University of California, Berkeley Wellness Letter.* Copyright © by Health Letter Associates, 1991. Page 55 Table 3.1 Reprinted from the American Lung Association. Page 58 Reprinted by permission of *Wall Street Journal.* Copyright © 1989 by Dow Jones & Company, Inc. All rights reserved worldwide. Page 61 Reprinted from the American Lung Association. Page 68 From *Design for a Livable Planet: How You Can Help Clean Up the Environment,* by J. Naar. Copyright © 1990 by J. Naar. Reprinted by permission of HarperCollins Publishers. Page 79 Reprinted from *American Health,* copyright © 1989 by M. Klockenbrink. Page 80 Reprinted with permission from the March/April 1991 issue of *Garbage* magazine, Brooklyn, New York. Page 84 From *Saving the Earth* by Will Steger and Jon Bowermaster. Copyright © 1990 by Byron Preiss Visual Publications and Will Steger and Jon Bowermaster. Reprinted with permission of Alfred A. Knopf, Inc. Page 91 Reprinted with permission from the January/February 1991 issue of *Garbage* magazine, Brooklyn, New York. Page 96 Reprinted courtesy of William L. Rathje. Page 99 From *Our Earth, Ourselves* by Ruth Caplan. © 1990 by Environmental Action, Inc. Used by permission of Bantam Books, a division of Bantam Doubleday Dell Publishing Group, Inc. Page 100 Reprinted with permission from *Science News,* the weekly newsmagazine of science. Copyright © 1988 by Science Service, Inc. Page 104 From *Design for a Livable Planet: How You Can Help Clean Up the Environment,* by J. Naar. Copyright © 1990 by J. Naar. Reprinted by permission of HarperCollins Publishers. Page 116 Reprinted with permission from *Healthline.*